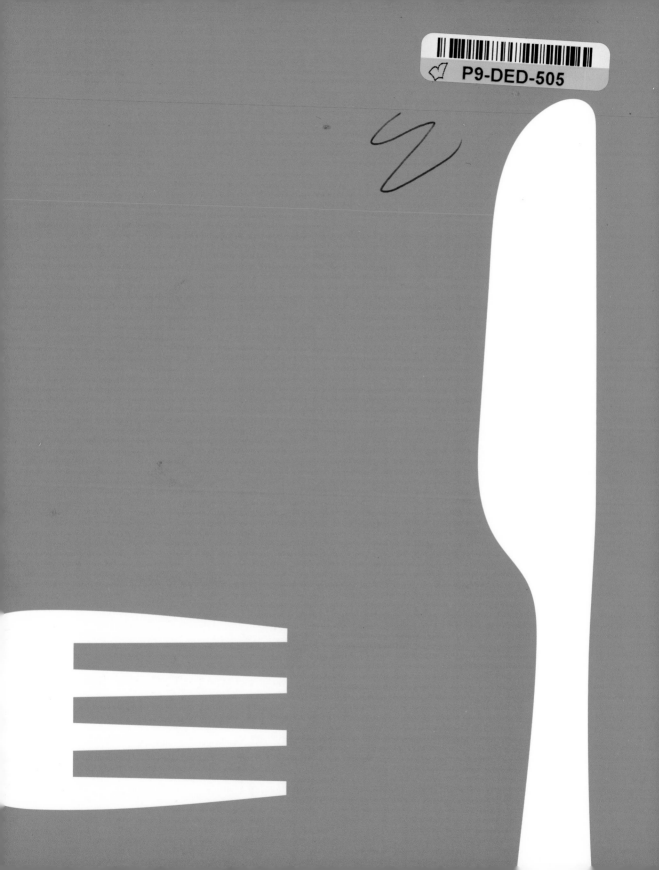

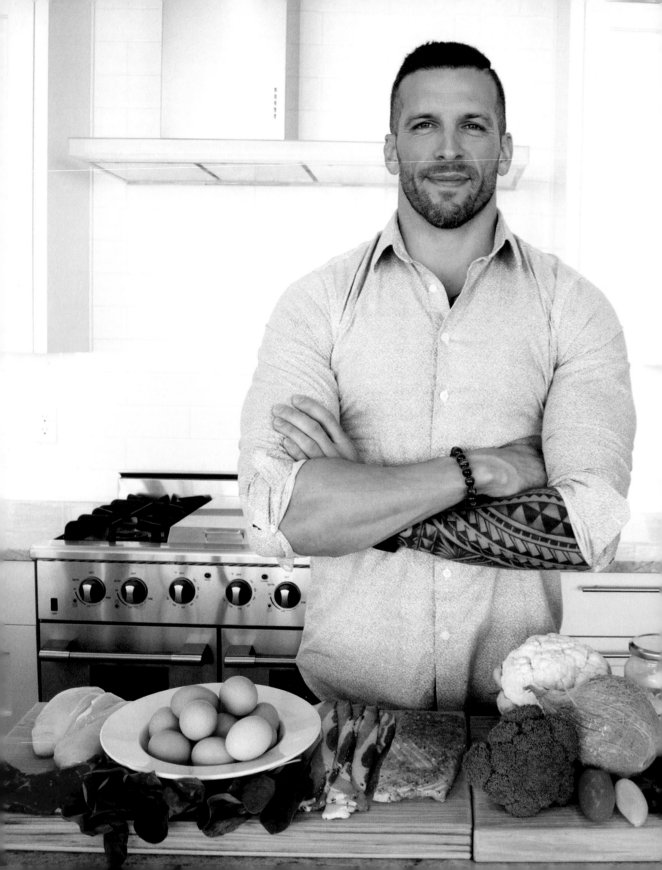

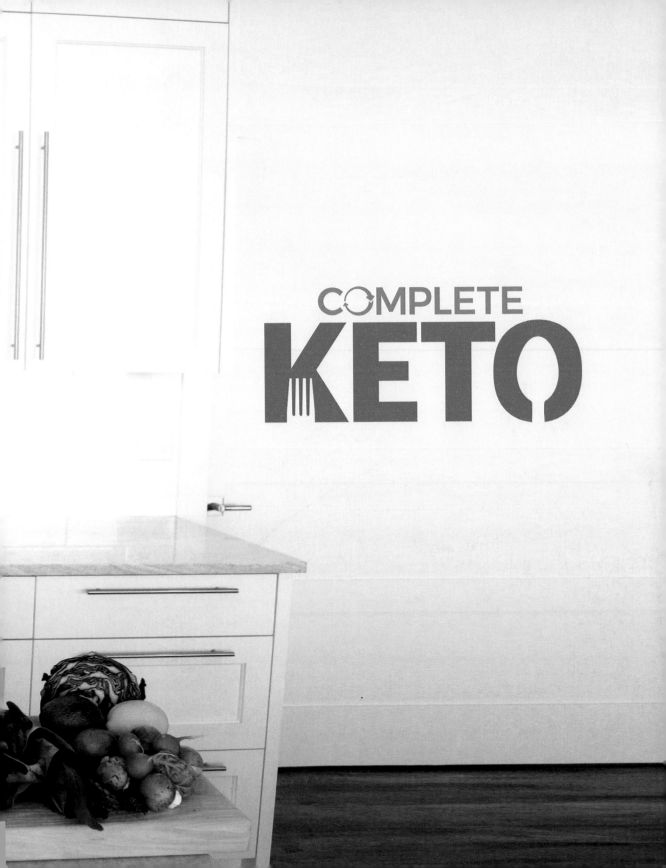

Also by DREW MANNING

Fit2Fat2Fit

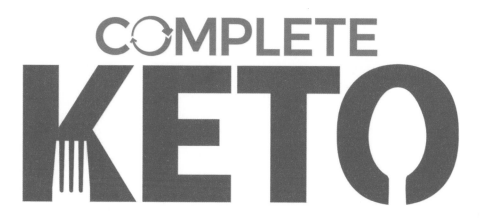

COMPLETE KETO

a guide to transforming
your body and your mind for life

DREW MANNING

HAY HOUSE, INC.

Carlsbad, California · New York City
London · Sydney · New Delhi

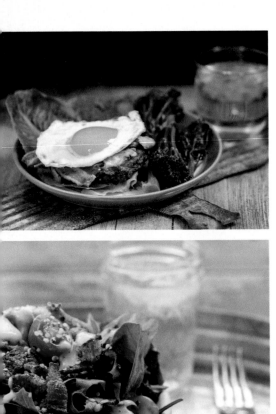

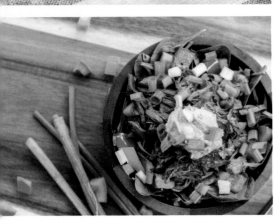

Published in the United States by:
Hay House, Inc.: www.hayhouse.com®

Published in Australia by:
Hay House Australia Pty. Ltd.: www.hayhouse.com.au

Published in the United Kingdom by:
Hay House UK, Ltd.: www.hayhouse.co.uk

Published in India by:
Hay House Publishers India: www.hayhouse.co.in

Cover and interior design: Charles McStravick
Exercise photos: Lyman Winn, L1quid Studios
Recipe photos: Bethers Photography
Photo of Drew on pages ii–iii: Adri Freeman, Adri Freeman Photography and Design
Photos of Drew on page xxii and page 344: Lyman Winn, L1quid Studios
Infographic images: Michael Roddy

Library of Congress Cataloging-in-Publication Data

Names: Manning, Drew, author.
Title: Complete keto : a guide to transforming your body and your mind for life / Drew Manning.
Description: Carlsbad, California : Hay House Inc., [2019]
Identifiers: LCCN 2018049663| ISBN 9781401956264 (hardback) | ISBN 9781401956288 (Ebook) | ISBN 9781401956271 (audiobook)
Subjects: LCSH: Ketogenic diet. | Low-carbohydrate diet--Recipes. | Reducing diets--Recipes. | BISAC: HEALTH & FITNESS / Weight Loss. | HEALTH & FITNESS / Diets.
Classification: LCC RC374.K46 M36 2019 | DDC 641.5/6383--dc23 LC record available at https://lccn.loc.gov/2018049663

Hardcover ISBN: 978-1-4019-5626-4
E-book ISBN: 978-1-4019-5628-8
Audiobook ISBN: 978-1-4019-5627-1

10 9 8 7 6 5 4 3 2 1
1st edition, February 2019

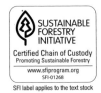

SUSTAINABLE FORESTRY INITIATIVE
Certified Chain of Custody
Promoting Sustainable Forestry
www.sfiprogram.org
SFI-01268

SFI label applies to the text stock

PRINTED IN THE UNITED STATES OF AMERICA

I want to dedicate this book to my

two beautiful daughters, Kale'a and Kiana,

who are my rock, my joy, and my purpose in this life.

I have the blessing and honor to be called their dad

and will be eternally grateful for them.

Strong fathers. Strong daughters.

CONTENTS

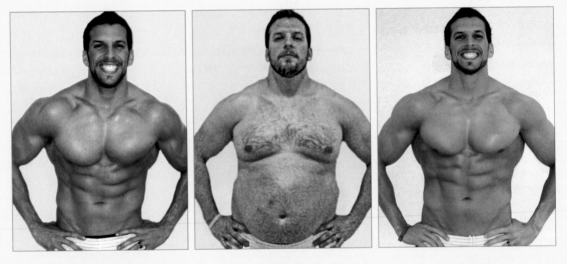

BEFORE   **DURING**   **AFTER**

INTRODUCTION

Nobody cares how much you know, until they know how much you care.

These are words I have lived by ever since I did my Fit2Fat2Fit journey, which put me on the *New York Times* bestseller list—and forever transformed the way I thought about helping people change.

What I learned on that journey was that you can have all the scientific knowledge and expertise in the world to help everyone achieve their weight loss goals, but none of that physical stuff matters unless you know how to relate to the people you're trying to help. This wisdom is where my next journey, Complete Keto, begins.

Most people know me as the Fit2Fat2Fit guy, the trainer who had this crazy idea to spend six months gaining 75 pounds and then lose it in another six months so I could better help my clients with their weight loss goals. You may have seen photos or television interviews with me at my highest weight—there

was even a meme of me going around for a while! I wrote a best-selling book chronicling my journey where I talked about how I learned way more about the mental and emotional aspects of weight loss than I did the physical. Appearing on national television and making the list were awesome experiences, but what most people don't know about me is that during that time, when everything seemed to be going great for me, I was also going through another big life transformation: my life as I knew it was falling apart.

You see, I grew up Mormon, which can be a very strict religion, and my perception was that I was never good enough. I believed

I was a failure because I had weaknesses, and if I couldn't be perfect, I wanted to *appear* perfect on the outside. I didn't want to talk about my weaknesses because I didn't want people to see me as a failure. It was a never-ending cycle of feeling shame, hiding my weakness, and striving for perfection so that people would like me and I would be worthy of being loved. This eventually broke me as a man. My marriage of 10 years ended, and that broke me too because I thought I would be a failure for the rest of my life. This was all during my Fit2Fat2Fit journey, where I appeared on TV shows like *Dr. Oz, The Tonight Show with Jay Leno,* and many others, and it seemed that at just the moment when I looked the most successful to the world—and when my life was the most public it had ever been—on the inside everything was breaking down.

Two things saved me. One was learning about the power of vulnerability and owning your story, which I got from working with a life coach and reading Brené Brown's amazing books. The other was keto. Yes, keto. Keto opened my eyes to *living optimally*: to mental clarity and amazing cognitive function, and to peak hormonal, gut, and emotional functioning.

Before keto, I looked great on the outside: in shape, eating healthy, and having all this success. But inside I was struggling with self-hate and feeling sluggish throughout the day because I was stressed out. I could fake it and get by, but more and more I noticed myself forgetting little details: people's names, where my car keys were, what I was supposed to be doing. I'd get sidetracked by my phone, or in the middle of a conversation suddenly find that I was wandering and couldn't remember my train of thought.

I first started on my keto journey after listening to a podcast where I learned the science behind it and heard the story of a man named Dr. Dom D'Agostino who, after a seven-day fast, deadlifted 500 pounds for 10 reps and 1 rep at 585 pounds. Doesn't that sound unreal—and super intriguing? After I asked some of my most trusted health and fitness friends, the science of what made this feat possible sounded legit. Were the results? Being the self-experimenter I am, I thought: Why not give this a try? I was curious to put my body to the test. So I decided to make a commitment and go all in; I'd do a 60-day 100 percent strict ketogenic diet, testing my blood ketone levels and everything.

And that's where I was converted. During those 60 days, two things ultimately sold me on keto. The first is that I found I was no longer a slave to food all the time. I wasn't as hungry, and so I didn't feel chained to the kitchen or to my body's cravings—and my emotional attachments to food were no longer a drain on me either. Before keto, I would eat six to seven small meals a day, and even though I'd always hit an afternoon slump, I thought that was what was best for my metabolism. I felt if I had to go two to three hours between meals I would lose all my muscle mass and my metabolism would slow down, so I was constantly prepping food and bringing Tupperware containers with me everywhere. On the keto diet, I was eating only one to two times per day and feeling so much more alert. Plus, my workouts were phenomenal.

The second thing that sold me on keto was the mental clarity. I had never experienced more mental clarity in my life. My cognitive function dramatically improved. It was like night and day compared to before. My brain was so much sharper. I felt on fire all the time. I could focus on tasks so much more intensely that I could get more work done far more efficiently. I could be doing speaking engagements up on stage, podcasting, writing blog posts, being an entrepreneur and a dad, and not lose my mental edge.

What keto did for my mental clarity and brain cognition helped me to see my body and my physical state of being more clearly, and this carried over into the mental, emotional, and spiritual realms as well. All those powerful concepts I was learning from Brené Brown and other personal development books and from my life coach were life-changing, but keto was the starting point for me to really understand and embody that wisdom—which helped me become a more complete human all around. I felt awake, alive, and in charge of my body, mind, and spirit.

I came to see that I had the power to change my perception, which meant I could change my story. I saw that I was in control of my own happiness. Not anybody else. Not any outside factors or sources. My happiness came from within. As Brown writes, "When we deny our stories, they define us. When we own our stories, we get to write a brave new ending."[1] Once keto helped me flip that switch and realize the power I had, I could own my life. I could write my own brave new ending. I could be authentically me and I didn't have to live my life constantly trying to please other people.

I went from fighting brain fog and struggling to focus on everyday tasks to having pure mental clarity, the capacity to focus intensely and control my thoughts and wandering mind. You've heard of the mind-body connection, right? The interdependent relationship between your body and mind means that better functioning of one will improve the other. My high-performing brain now gives me that endless energy we see in kids and so desperately want to bottle. Keto is my "energy in a bottle."

I also went from seeing everything in extreme black and white, paralyzed by what other people thought of me, paralyzed that they would find out I wasn't perfect and that I had weaknesses, to a deep understanding that it's okay to love yourself and okay to be vulnerable. When you feel optimal and your thinking is clear, you're empowered to own your story. There is so much power in living an authentic life for you that isn't dependent on what other people think of you.

You've probably read about this weird-sounding food plan that's all the rage these days, but the truth is that keto is actually a very old diet—it's been used since the turn of the century as a therapeutic diet for people suffering from seizures, and researchers believe that long before that, our early ancestors likely lived a very ketogenic lifestyle. What is new is the way I combine my unique meal and workout plan with a total mind/body/spirit transformation that teaches you how to live an optimal life. That's what Complete Keto means to me: an optimal and complete body-mind transformation.

THE BENEFITS OF COMPLETE KETO

How different would your life be if you woke up with tons of energy, had a sharp-as-a-tack mind, and felt full of motivation and ready to go for hours on end? How liberated would you feel if you were no longer a slave to meal prep and food cravings, but instead could listen to your body tell you exactly what it needs and only what it needs to run efficiently? What would you do with that much energy, mental clarity, and free time?

The reason I advocate the keto diet isn't because it can give you six-pack abs, or help you shed excess weight fast, or keep you ripped and shredded 24/7. Yes, you can build muscle and lose fat on the keto diet. But to me, those are all bonuses. Perks. Welcome side effects of living a keto lifestyle. What it's really about for me is what it does for your life. The main reason I became hooked on keto and now am a huge proponent of this lifestyle is that keto gave my brain life. And it can do the same for you.

Do you know what it's like for small tasks to seem larger and more complicated than they are? To feel like your brain is shut off and won't turn on—or won't turn off when you need it to? Have you ever felt unable to fully focus on a task, or struggled with wandering thoughts?

What about going through your day feeling slow, as if you're treading through some invisible sludge, then being completely and totally exhausted by 2 P.M. and feeding wicked sugar cravings to help get you through? Or the frustration of not being able to recall words and phrases, or even forgetting things from your past that you used to remember so vividly?

Can you relate?

What if you knew you could feel mentally sharp all the time? Optimal. Not a slave to food, not having to eat every two to three hours, not feeling hangry (hungry + angry), with energy levels through the roof, a focused mind all day long, skin clear.

Here's the thing: we've been lied to as a society. For the past 50 years we've been taught that eating fat makes you fat and that fats are bad. Remember that food pyramid from grade school? Seven to 11 servings of grains per day; eat fats sparingly. The keto diet flips that on its head. The latest research is showing that fats are actually healthy for our bodies. In fact, they are a most efficient source of energy.

As a society we're on all kinds of medications for diseases and illnesses that have inflammation at their core; we're tired, we're wired, our joints ache, and we struggle to lose weight. The ketogenic diet reduces inflammation in the body and brain and increases blood flow, which is why you'll have the sharpest and clearest mental abilities of your life with keto. It's also why so many people are able to get off their medications on keto: get to the root of inflammation and your body will function optimally. With the keto lifestyle you're fully fueling your body and brain, so you'll find you don't have to eat as much to feel satiated and you won't be hungry in between meals, which means you can spend less time planning meals, cooking, and prepping food and more time enjoying your life. You never feel like you're starving and you rarely feel you have to snack (although there are great keto snacks if you do!). Instead, your body will naturally remind you when it's time to eat. You'll find you can work out, work all day, play with the kids, and not ever feel sluggish.

The keto lifestyle can help create a brain that is stronger, works faster, activates untapped energy, and helps your body operate optimally. When you get your brain on board, the body follows. That's when you start seeing those results so many people talk about when doing keto: shedding body fat quickly, reduction in joint pain, sleeping like a baby. (Better than a baby, actually, because babies sleep like crap.) You stop being dependent on caffeine, sugar, carbs, and other stimulants, and you just feel open and on. When your mind is clear, sharp, and focused, you become the highest performing version of yourself, someone who has all the energy, health, and brainpower to create a life you love. When you feel fantastic, you do fantastic things.

I've worked with a wide range of people—athletes, CEOs, stay-at-home moms, celebrities, coaches, trainers, construction workers, and entrepreneurs among them—and I've seen them all utilize the ketogenic diet to enhance their cognitive function and optimize their brain performance. It's helped them perform at higher levels with great clarity of mind no matter how they fill their days, and it's giving them powerful reserves of energy with which to exceed their fitness and health goals. Keto is helping them become a better, faster, smarter, and leaner version of themselves—and they still get to eat delicious, filling food.

Complete Keto isn't a temporary crash diet; it's a lifestyle program you can use to create a better life for yourself. I believe it because it worked for me, helping me transition from a very difficult time to a life that now feels authentic, full, and happy in body, mind, and spirit. I wrote this book to teach you everything I know and to give you all the tools required for your success.

It's *your* turn now. Now is the time to own your story, take control of your life, totally change your perception of what health is supposed to look like on your body, and be the best version of you that you can possibly be.

COMPLETE KETO: THE BEST VERSION OF YOU

For so long the health and fitness industry has been dominated by bodybuilder magazines, celebrities on TV, and, more recently, Instagram models. We see these images everywhere we go—on billboards, social media, commercials, magazines, reality TV, and more—and we think that needs to be our version of healthy and fit. What if that's just not true? What if the truth is that that televised version of healthy and fit is not for everybody? We live in a society that's all about choices and yet we're all striving for a one-size-fits-all body, with six-pack abs, tiny waistlines, and cut biceps. Does that make any sense at all? NOPE.

Complete Keto is here to show you that what it really all comes down to is you living your *optimal life* and that there's a parallel between the physical journey and the mental, emotional, and spiritual journey. Just like I needed to learn that all things are not black or white—that being vulnerable or having weaknesses and struggles didn't mean I wasn't worthy of being loved—we all need to learn that we can love ourselves and our bodies on the journey to health rather than waiting to be happy until we reach [fill in the blank with your ideal weight]. My Complete Keto program will empower you to discover what health and fitness look like on *you*. With two phases, including a unique mind-body-spirit-focused 30-day keto program and a second phase that covers everything you need to know about doing keto long-term, I'm going to help you realize that *your* version of healthy does not need to be defined by what you see in the media. You are not a failure if you don't achieve instafamous status.

This is so much more than a 30-day diet book that will help you lose weight. Yes, you will lose weight on my plan, and yes, you'll have more mental clarity and more energy, too. But Complete Keto is also an invitation to a true lifestyle change—a physical, mental, emotional, spiritual transformation. I know that the hook is the physical part—this keto diet is awesome, you'll feel amazing, you'll experience all the physical benefits that you've heard everyone rave about, and I'm a keto expert who's put together my absolutely best program for you! All that is true. At the same time, I want you to be surprised that this is so much more than you thought it would be. My goal is not just to have you feeling physically great, but to empower you to take control of your life.

Take my friend Anne, for example. When she first came to my program she was beyond frustrated. Her friends all seemed able to lose weight while she felt completely stuck. Every diet she tried, she'd lose a couple pounds and then gain them right back again. Her health

was suffering. She was on a steady diet of medications for blood pressure, cholesterol, and thyroid. Her energy was low, and she was struggling with very low self-esteem.

Within two weeks of being on my program, Anne let me know that for her keto is a complete lifestyle change. She loved how fast she lost weight. That was a strong motivator, for sure. More than that, though, she *loves* that keto doesn't feel like a diet. "If it's a diet," she says, "I'd stop eventually." But keto—it's not just a diet. It's changed the way she sees her whole life. She eats food she loves, enjoys meals out with friends, and even has a blast picking out new clothes as her body changes. She feels confident in her body. She no longer needs all the medications. She has energy and clarity. With keto, she told me, she gets to live longer *and* enjoy the journey. This is exactly the kind of body/mind/spirit transformation I hear every day from people on my programs, and it's the heart of Complete Keto.

It's important to me that when you go on this keto journey you are supported with great food, great workouts, *and* tons of emotional support so you aren't just eating keto, you're healing any emotional or spiritual obstacles that may come up along the way. That's what makes it a lifestyle and not just a diet. My program isn't just a list of what to eat and what to avoid; it's a whole new approach to fitness that helps you overcome the guilt and shame so deeply associated with food, weight, and health in our society so that you can get to *your* best health without apology.

So let me state right here in the beginning: you are not a number on a scale. Losing weight and achieving your health goals aren't as easy as black and white. Frankly, it's not even as easy as flipping a switch and doing the things you know you're "supposed" to. It's hard. It's way more mental and emotional than it is just physical. However, I learned that if you can overcome the mental and emotional challenges, you'll be well on your way to making this program a lifestyle rather than just another diet.

My goal is to give you all the tools you need to make this into a lifestyle change so that you don't just lose the weight and gain it back, but help you realize that it's not even just about weight loss at all. You'll be able to focus on the process and creating healthy habits and let the results (weight loss and physical appearance) take care of themselves. I don't even care if you don't do my plan; I just want you to feel healthy and happy. In fact, I encourage you to think of me as a trusted guide and *you* as the expert on *your* health. I am a keto expert, and I've walked the walk, but you know your health journey best. Consult your doctor about specifics related to your own health, including conditions like type 1 diabetes, liver disease, thyroid, and more—I've even included some support for talking to your doctor about keto in the resources section at the back of the book. I don't want to be just another voice telling you what to do. I want to empower you to be your own self-experimenter and to find *your* optimal. I want to give you tons of help and hope and a great program you can use as a stepping stone in your journey to feeling amazing, because you're worth it. Fight for your health.

There's so much more to you than what your body looks like and how much you weigh. You have so much more to offer this world other than your body fat percentage. Don't base your self-worth on your relationship with gravity. Focus on health and healthy habits first and the process, and let weight loss and the results be a byproduct of living that healthy lifestyle over time. Complete Keto will empower you to do just that.

ABOUT DREW AND THIS BOOK

My journey to own my life, my story, and my happiness led me down a path of personal development and coaching people on so much more than just a diet program. In 2009 I started out as a National Academy of Sports Medicine (NASM)-certified trainer working with clients one-on-one—from there I embarked on my Fit2Fat2Fit journey in 2011 seeking to better understand why clients struggled so much to lose weight. I learned from my Fit2Fat2Fit experience that empathy and understanding are far more important motivators than knowing the right form for doing burpees. This profoundly changed me as a trainer because it showed me that while one-on-one coaching is important, what really gave me meaning was to have large-scale impact and change the idea of one-size-fits-all fitness altogether.

Today I work with clients in the form of large social media groups so that rather than one person training one person at a time I can create safe spaces where everybody helps each other out. My team and I give people all the tools they need to transform physically: fitness, nutrition, and constant support for any nutrition and workout questions that may come up.

But in my groups people also get the mental and emotional coaching they need to motivate and inspire them so they know they're worth it. It's a safe place to post about failures, to ask "dumb" questions, to share progress photos where you're not going to be judged or put down—where instead you'll have people cheering you on, lifting you up, and motivating you to push harder than you would on your own. And you're able to pay it forward by giving others support and motivating them. I'm proud to say that all six of Tony Robbins's six basic human needs—certainty, uncertainty, feeling significant, connection/love, progress or happiness found by setting and achieving goals, and giving back or making an impact—are being met in my Facebook groups.

All my experiences have taught me that transformation is more mental and emotional than we think. Of course you need to know about the principles of keto, what to eat, and how to move, but there are additional pieces to the puzzle, and you need all of them to complete the picture. My main focus is helping people overcome their mental and emotional challenges, and these groups are how I do it, by listening to your real struggles and cultivating a safe space for you to share your struggles and your accomplishments—a place where there is no judgement, only support, love, encouragement, empathy, and respect.

I've written this book with the same philosophy I've used to create my groups: in it you'll find a judgement-free zone and lots of love and encouragement. It's got everything you need to know about what the ketogenic diet is, how it works and why, and lots of tips, tricks, and hacks for incorporating it into your life in a way that works best for you, plus all the mental and emotional support you'll need to make keto a true life transformation.

The book is organized into six parts. Parts 1 and 2 will answer all your questions about what keto is, why it works, and what's so great about it so that you're set up to embark on this journey with everything you need. In Part 1 I'll dispel common myths about keto, lay out the keto macros, and outline what to eat and what to avoid, with a special shout-out to women and vegetarians and vegans (veg*n for short) interested in keto. I also include my top hacks for overcoming mental and emotional obstacles with food. In Part 2 I get into the nitty gritty of getting started on keto: what being in "ketosis" means and how to test for it, how to avoid and deal with side effects, how to supplement, and how to stay keto while dining out and traveling. Lots of emotional support here as well.

Part 3 is phase one of my program, Complete Keto 30, or CK30. My plan is what I call a "keto cleanse" that, while strict, sets you up for wins the whole way through by getting your body efficient at living keto as quickly as possible so you can reap the benefits of weight loss, reduced inflammation, and improved mental clarity. You'll find 30 days of meal plans, my workout program, meditations and affirmations to support you mentally and spiritually during the cleanse, my advice on 24-hour fasting, and a sample veg*n meal plan.

Part 4 is phase two of my program, where I give you options for going beyond the "cleanse" phase and incorporating keto into your life in the best way for *you*. Unlike all other keto programs, I break my program into these two parts because before you can think about doing keto long-term, I want to help you get into a state of ketosis so that your body becomes a fat burning machine! And then in phase two, I'll help you make the best use of your now fat-adapted body so that you can continue to make progress over time. Part 4 also includes my final words of motivation and encouragement as you head out on your own. Part 5 explains and illustrates how to do the exercises in the workout program—the basic movements as well as modifications that work for any body. Part 6 might be my favorite part: dozens of delicious recipes you'll use to transform your body and mind!

Throughout the book I'll share my favorite groups, apps, and other resources to help make your keto journey the best it can be—and check out the Resources section all the way at the end for even more support. You'll also see many powerful "before" and "after" photos and testimonials throughout the book, but I ask you to keep in mind that the "after" can just as easily be titled "during" or "continuing on" or "moving forward still." The term "after" feels like you're done, but in this plan there is no finish line. In fact, many of the people featured in this book asked for more time to submit new "after" photos because they continued to change so much while waiting for the book to come out! It's important to track your progress, but remember we are always a work *in* progress—and that's a beautiful thing.

You'll hear me talk throughout the book about your "why," and that's more important to me than your "after." What I mean by your "why" is figuring out why you want to get healthy and optimize your life. What's your motivation? It should be a why that is bigger than just yourself and bigger than wanting to look good or be thin—that's a cool goal and it might motivate you for a season, but what happens to your motivation when you lose the weight? Think back to the six basic needs I mentioned above—happiness is *progress*. That's why even some celebrities who seem like they have anything anyone could ever want can still get depressed. When there's nothing else to give you meaning and motivation, you lose your sense of progress and purpose. Finding a why means committing to progress in life and letting go of the idea of a finish line.

The heart of this book, and all my work, is the realization that you are worth it. With Complete Keto I'm here to show you that it really all comes down to living an optimal life—and that you deserve it and it is achievable. The combination of my unique two-part keto program with plenty of mental, emotional, and spiritual support makes total transformation possible.

Does that seem almost overwhelming or too good to believe? Don't worry; you won't be doing it alone. Because you picked up this book, you have me and thousands of others that have walked this path. I'm not going to shame you or yell at you to put down that food or get your ass off the couch—I'm going to walk beside you to give you all the tools you need to succeed and a strong dose of understanding, encouragement, and empathy when times get tough. I'm going to empower you to live your most energized, healthy life, all while enjoying delicious, simple whole foods. You ready to get started?

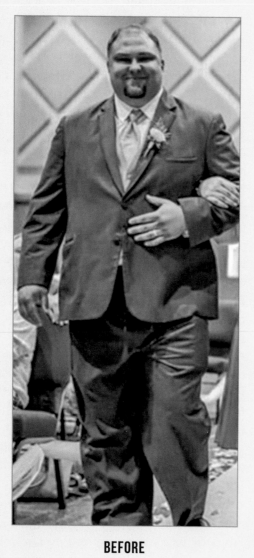

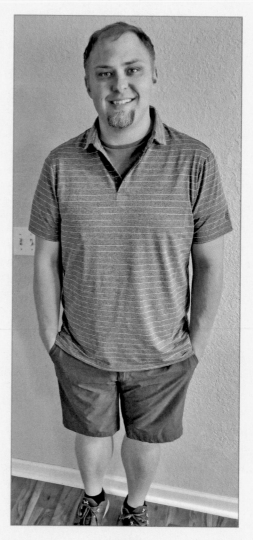

BEFORE   **AFTER**

TYLER ROBBINS

AFTER YEARS OF BEING DOWN ABOUT MY WEIGHT AND MAKING EXCUSES FOR MYSELF the heavier I got, I had an honest talk with myself. I am someone's husband and dad. I owe it to them to be the best person I can be. My life isn't just my own, my life impacts so many others. I want to be able to be active with my daughters and be able to do fun stuff with my wife without feeling exhausted or unable to because of my size.

I spent so many years saying, "I won't let myself hit this weight." When I hit that weight, I said it again, "I won't let myself hit this next weight." It became toxic toward me. I looked into several diets and weight loss methods including surgery. I didn't want to put our family through the costs of a major elective surgery like that. My biggest issue with food has been addiction. I always worried about when I would eat and what I would eat. It consumed my thoughts far too often and it made me realize just how often I was eating.

Upon looking into diets I stumbled across Fit2Fat2Fit. After looking at model after model telling me how to look like them, I saw Drew Manning. While he is in incredible shape, he actually proved how you can lose the weight by putting on a whole bunch. I don't see the South Beach models doing that. It resonated with me when I read about how you can become fat-adapted and the fat satiates you and you don't feel hungry. This was my primary concern, trying to get that little demon inside of me to stop telling me I'm hungry. Once I got to know the program I took a day to think it over.

After consideration I started Keto on his Jumpstart plan. I decided to challenge myself. My challenge was starting the first week of December. I told myself, if I can stay strong through Christmas and New Year's, nothing can stop me. The second week of January hit and I had to replace my belt. The one I had been using was on the hole second to last from the end. In February I had to replace my dress pants for work and shirts. In April I had to replace all of my shorts for spring. Here we are in May. The belt I replaced is at the last hole. I bought it when the second to last from the end was comfortable. Now I'm at the last hole and will be replacing it soon.

I can honestly say I have not had one single bite that was cheating. I have been fine not eating at events where the food was not something I could have. I did this by using my why as my strength and my accountability. I told myself early on when I felt weak, "This cookie isn't worth ruining what you've done so far. Your girls need you to stay strong." I am happily at 80 pounds lost since the first of December and still counting. I had allowed myself to get to a weight I'm extremely disgusted with, however, I am now at the same weight I was in high school 15 years ago. I feel incredible, my knees don't hurt anymore. I have a pop in my step again. Stairs aren't something I dread. This was the best decision of my life because it has given me my life back.

This program works, but only if you dedicate yourself to this. If you attack it as I did, you WILL succeed. It's a journey, not a sprint. This is a commitment and needs to be treated that way. This isn't a "Well, I'll cheat today and make up for it tomorrow." That's not how this works. If you're at that point in your life, this isn't for you. If you're where I was, looking to make a change and willing to take it on 100 percent, you will look back months from now and wish you would have found it sooner. Join Keto and good luck!

— TYLER ROBBINS

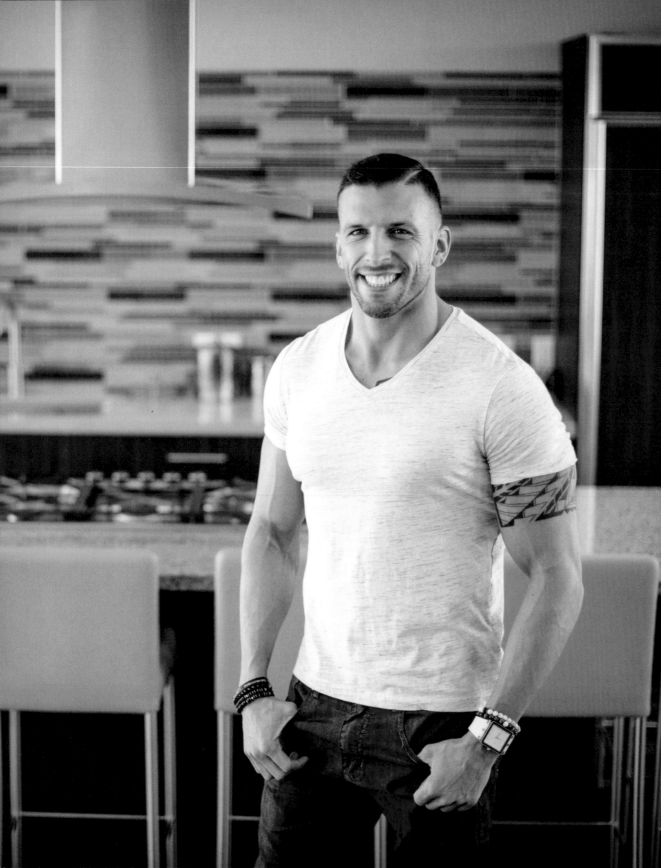

PART 1

COMPLETE KETO 101

I know from experience that this is hard. Changing your lifestyle, changing your mind-set, changing old habits—it can seem impossible. And it's going to be really hard for a lot of people. But I'm here to hold your hand and walk you through this and let you know that it's worth it to continue fighting for your health and it IS possible. Some diet programs will tell you that dieting isn't hard. They take a tough love approach to kicking your butt into shape. It's only a 14- or 30-day program, after all.

But you know what? It is hard. It's hard to change your relationship to food; it's hard to face things about your body and your health that you'd rather keep hidden. I've been where you are: wanting to lose weight and feel better in my life, longing for more energy to play with my kids, but also crying over the loss of my beloved Cinnamon Toast Crunch and evenings spent vegging out on the couch.

I talked a lot in my first book, *Fit2Fat2Fit*, about how I once thought of fitness as a summit you reach—a mountain you climb— with fit people on the top and everyone else at the bottom, overwhelmed at the thought of needing to climb so far. You probably know this feeling well: fear of the sheer size of that mountain, all the "get slim fast" promises spinning in your head as you fantasize about quicker and easier ways to traverse those miles. It was through my own journey from Fit2Fat2Fit that I learned that there are way more shades of gray in the mix.

The problem with most diet plans is that they give you only 14 or 30 days of support without addressing the lifestyle change that needs to happen. They see things only in black and white, fat or fit. They only help you get closer to the top of that mountain. Then what? You're just standing at the top like, cool, I made it. The truth is, there is no finish line. This journey does not end when you lose the weight you want. Weight loss is just the beginning. I don't just want to help you achieve your weight loss goals—I want to revolutionize your whole life and help you see yourself, your body, from a totally different and healthier perspective.

To do that, you need both a program and support for making holistic lifestyle changes. I'm going to give you that. Why Complete Keto? Because with Complete Keto you begin to learn what made you emotionally dependent on food and how to overcome that while working on a better version of yourself physically, psychologically, and even spiritually. With my program you forge a deeper connection to *yourself* rather than with food. You come back to you: your natural energy, your natural clarity, your optimal well-being.

WHAT IS THE KETOGENIC DIET?

Most people think keto is just watered-down Paleo, or bacon cheeseburgers without the bun. Fair enough—a ketogenic (keto) diet *is* a high-fat, moderate-protein, and low-carb diet; BUT it's also a comprehensive, holistic approach to optimal functioning and health.

So what is keto really?

The purpose of a ketogenic diet is to get you into a state of *ketosis*. On a very basic level, ketosis is the natural metabolic state that your body goes into when there is no glucose—aka carbs—available to burn for energy.

Your body needs fuel to keep your brain, organs, *everything*, functioning. Most people are walking around burning glucose for fuel. But our bodies are designed to run on two different types of fuel. One is glucose, which is what most of our foods—breads, pastas, rices, grains, potatoes, cereals—are converted to. And the other fuel source? Ketones, which are produced by breaking down fatty acids. By restricting carbohydrates, you trigger your body's backup fuel burning system and reprogram your metabolism to burn your stored body fat for fuel instead.

What this means is that our body breaks down fatty acids—the stored fat in our bodies—and the liver converts them to these awesome things called "ketones." Then ketones become the primary energy source for our brain, muscles, and organs so they can function properly.

Ketones are just a different type of fuel source for your body. They also happen to be a more efficient fuel source. Why? Because glucose is a fast-burning energy source and ketones are a slow, sustained energy source that our bodies can run on for a long time.

Think of it this way: You have a fire going. It's nice and cozy. But the fire starts to dwindle a bit and you're trying to impress your kids with your pyrotechnic ability. You want a roaring fire. What to do? If you throw paper or lighter fluid on the fire, that will certainly

VISUALIZING KETONES

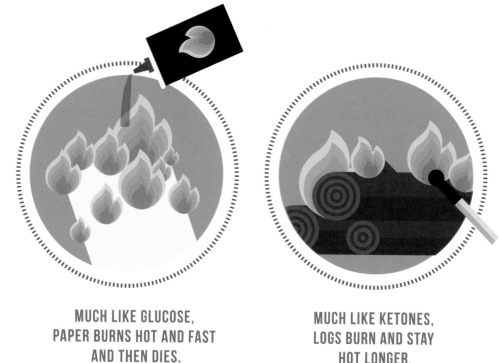

MUCH LIKE GLUCOSE, PAPER BURNS HOT AND FAST AND THEN DIES.

MUCH LIKE KETONES, LOGS BURN AND STAY HOT LONGER.

give you an increase in the flames—but only for a short period of time before the flames return to their normal state. In the same way, you drink an energy drink or eat a donut when you feel an afternoon slump coming on. Will you get a burst of energy? Sure. Will your body sustain that energy? Nope.

Ketones, on the other hand, are the logs or the coal of the fire that stay lit for a long period of time. When you're burning ketones, you're going to burn fat for fuel and you're giving your brain and your whole body a highly efficient, long-lasting source of energy. Sweet.

To put it into perspective: Your body can only store up to about 3,000 calories of glucose at one time, which most people burn through in a day or two. Or you can tap into about 30,000 calories of stored fat for fuel. In other words, your body can run a long time on ketones. I'm talking about a very efficient fuel source; I'm talking about a metabolic reset that turns you into an optimally functioning human. When you're burning fat for fuel, you won't just get an energy boost, you'll be able to maintain that energy long-term. That's good for your body *and* your brain.

This state of being in ketosis is a natural one. It is NOT an unhealthy state to be in. Our bodies have this built-in backup system to keep us alive and well when food is scarce. That may seem strange in our modern society where most of us can probably go to Walmart or Whole Foods and get any food we want any time of the day, any day of the week (#FoodOnDemand), but our ancestors probably had to go days at a time without any food as part of the natural rhythm of hunting and gathering. If we didn't have this backup system, humankind probably wouldn't have been able to survive and I wouldn't be here writing this book. Yet here I am. And because of this backup system, if we stopped eating today, we wouldn't die tomorrow. I promise you. You're not going to die from one day of no food. You might feel like it when you're hangry. Been there. But you won't. Your body will simply use up all the glucose it's storing for fuel and then the backup system will kick in and start burning stored fat for fuel, and you'll be in a state of ketosis.

Your body can burn only so much glucose; the rest gets stored as fat. For our ancestors, this system worked in balance. They had natural ebbs and flows in their food availability. For us, in a society in which food is not only *not* scarce but in fact overabundant and overwhelmingly made up of processed carbohydrates, which admittedly taste freaking delicious, it's not surprising we see obesity at all-time high levels, as well as sluggishness and mental exhaustion. It's no wonder most of us are struggling to meet our weight loss goals no matter what program we choose,

or that we feel that late afternoon crash that often ends in an anxious or burnt-out feeling by the end of the day. The problem is that the modern diet and modern weight loss regimens aren't fully engaging the amazing power of our body's systems. Instead of optimizing the body's systems, they're overloading and slowing them down.

There are two ways to get into ketosis: One is to stop eating. Fasting. Like our ancestors. This is really hard to do, because we've been eating three meals a day for 30, 40, 50 years. Our whole life. So to stop eating is not fun for a lot of people. But a way to hack that is with the ketogenic diet, which is the second way to get into ketosis, where your body is getting about 70 percent of its calories from fat, about 25 percent from protein, and about 5 percent from carbohydrates. Eating this way forces your body into a state of ketosis, in which you use fat as fuel.

In a nutshell, the ketogenic diet is your body's backup system. Your body can't convert fat into glucose, but your body can convert excess protein and carbohydrates into glucose. When you limit your protein and carbohydrate intake your body runs out of glucose on which to run, so it's forced to produce ketones, which are a very efficient fuel source for our bodies.

So ketosis is the state that you achieve when your body breaks down ketones (fat) for energy rather than running on the glucose from carbohydrates. You *want* to get into ketosis. You *want* to start to burn your body fat for fuel. A keto diet is not a diet that you can choose to go on and off at any point. It takes time for your body to adjust and go into this metabolic state known as ketosis. How long does this process take? It can take anywhere from two to seven days, depending on your body type, activity levels, and what you're eating. The goal of a ketogenic diet is not only to achieve ketosis, to switch your body from running on glucose to running on ketones, but to become what's called fat-adapted. When you are fat-adapted you fully harness the power of burning fat for fuel—and all the energy that brings—long-term. In a nutshell, you're very efficient at burning fat for fuel and you feel optimal . . . more optimal than you ever have.

And your brain? Well, your brain loves ketones as much as Beyoncé loves bedazzled bodysuits. (She does!) Well, actually, your brain loves ketones as much as it loves glucose—it's just that ketones provide your brain with really efficient fuel as well as neuroprotective benefits. In other words, the same clean energy that your body derives from burning ketones also fuels your brain really well.

You have thousands upon thousands upon thousands of calories stored in your body fat. By restricting carbs and prioritizing filling, whole-food sources of fat, your body is forced to tap into the calories from your body fat and burn that for muscle and brain fuel. Isn't that incredible? It's a total metabolic body reset that will have you thinking faster and sharper, enhancing your ability to focus your mind and get tasks done without procrastinating and living in brain fog. And you shed excess body fat in the process. Ain't nothing wrong with that!

MYTHS ABOUT KETO

The thought of purposely putting your body into a different metabolic state may seem scary or unnatural. I get that. Isn't biohacking our metabolism only the stuff of elite athletes, scientists, nerds, rich people, and Silicon Valley CEOs and not for, say, your average PTA parent? Fear may come up, too, because we've been sold a lie for so long about how fat is bad for us, for our waistlines and our hearts. As one person told me: "I've been on one diet or another since I was thirteen years old and the one thing they all have in common is the rule that fat is bad." I get questions all the time from people with all kinds of misconceptions about what keto is and isn't, so I wanted to take some time right from the start to address the most common myths about the keto lifestyle.

The truth is that ketosis is a natural and normal state for the body to be in, and more and more scientists, doctors, and researchers are showing how beneficial this lifestyle is every day.

In fact, when babies are born and eating only breast milk or formula, they are in a mild state of ketosis until we kick them out with that first bowl of rice cereal or mashed sweet potatoes. And do you know how efficient infants are at developing everything from their brains to their organs? Wicked efficient, my friend.

So let's dispel some of the top myths about the ketogenic diet:

MYTH #1:
All that fat will clog your arteries, raise your blood pressure, and give you a heart attack

This is the big myth about keto. The founding father of myths about keto, if you will. The myth that leads to all other myths. So let's really break this one down.

Yes, it's true that a lot of the older science showed that high fat in your diet caused clogged arteries and heart disease. But what those studies don't tell you is that they didn't factor in the number of carbs that were being consumed in those diets. Carbs are the problem, not fat.[1] If you take carbohydrates out of the equation, a high-fat diet is *not* associated with clogged arteries or heart disease. In fact, it's associated with *lower* inflammation and reduced weight, which is good in a lot of different ways.

Inflammation is the root cause of so much illness and disease—everything from dementia to obesity and, yup, you guessed it: heart disease, too. What leading researchers are finding is that the ketogenic diet is an absolute powerhouse when it comes to fighting inflammation, naturally and quickly lowering inflammation throughout the body.[2] Keto is like a five-time Olympic gold medalist of lowering inflammation. Get up on that podium and take a bow, keto.

But how can this be, you ask, when we were told for so long that fat was bad for us?

Not to sound like a conspiracy theorist, but those low-fat, low-cholesterol recommendations we'd been hearing about from the 1970s on (and that we all so dutifully believed)? Well, they were a result of food companies paying off doctors to say that low-fat, sugar-heavy foods are good for you. For real.

In 2017 we actually started to get clear and compelling evidence of this. We now know that the sugar industry spent (and still spends) a lot of time and money convincing us that there is no link between sugar and heart disease, cancer, and other health issues; and yet researchers found that as early as 1968 the Sugar Research Foundation itself had evidence connecting a high-sugar diet to increased risk of heart attack, stroke, and even bladder cancer.[3] Um, what?! But the industry halted the study as soon as those findings came in. Curious, am I right? What they did continue to fund, however, were studies that downplayed the connection between sugar consumption and blood-fat levels. So there's that.

The outcome of all this is that we were told for *decades* that fat caused weight gain and heart disease, and as a result we were fed mountains of low-fat, low-calorie, processed-sugar "diet" foods. Did this in any way decrease obesity rates? Nope. Did it decrease the rates of heart disease? Nope. In fact, it did quite the opposite.

Let's look at some numbers: In 1970 the obesity rates were less than 14 percent. As of 2016, 35.2 percent of the population was overweight, and 29.6 percent was obese. If our society continues this trend, our projected obesity and overweight rate will be 46 percent by 2030.[4]

As Jimmy Moore puts it, "In just the past few decades, the rates of obesity, diabetes, heart disease, and other chronic illnesses have

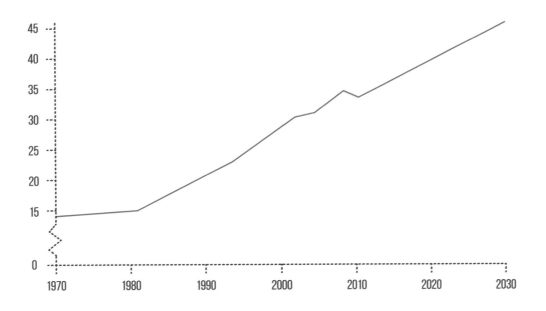

In 1970 the obesity rates were less than 14%. As of 2016, 35.2% of the population was overweight, and 29.6% are obese. If our society continues this trend our projected obesity & overweight rate will be 46% by 2030.

gotten considerably worse. And do you know what's most shocking about that? The spike in all these ailments coincides almost perfectly with the implementation of the government's Dietary Guidelines in 1980. Coincidence? I think not."[5] Same, Jimmy. Same.

We know now that inflammation is a major culprit in so many of our health issues—heart disease, obesity, autoimmune disease, and more—and we know that sugar, and not fat, is inextricably linked to inflammation. Some of the most well-respected researchers in the world are showing us that healthy, whole-food sources of fat are not only good for us, they're actually necessary for optimal functioning of our brains, hormones, and more. It's a major change in thinking, I know. But it's time to ditch the idea that fat is bad for us and embrace its inflammation-fighting abilities.

MYTH #2:
Your body needs glucose to function

Yes, your body does need some glucose to function. More specifically, your brain and liver need a *small* amount of glucose to function optimally. To be ridiculously specific: your brain can use about 120 grams of glucose a day to function—which translates to about 30 grams of carbohydrates. You will get some of that from the ketogenic diet because you will be consuming a minimal amount of carbohydrates. And the rest?

Here's an amazing thing about your body: it can and will produce its own glucose even if you are not consuming glucose. How? Through a process called gluconeogenesis, which is a fancy word for the process by which your body generates glucose from things that aren't carbohydrates, like protein for example.[6] So by eating minimal carbohydrates and no processed sugar, and through the process of gluconeogenesis, your body will still be able to produce the amount of glucose it needs to function off—and the rest of your body functions really well from ketones. Cool, right?

MYTH #3:
Keto is just Atkins repackaged

Fair enough: the notoriously low-carb Atkins diet is similar to Keto. But Atkins is low carb, high protein, and high fat while Keto is low carb, moderate protein, and high fat. What's the difference? The Atkins diet does work well for some people—I know a lot of bodybuilders who do a modified approach to Atkins/keto, and it works for them because they have a lot of muscle mass and are very active. However, when the average person consumes too much protein it can be converted to glucose (by that process I discussed above, called gluconeogenesis), and so lots of people end up feeling horrible on Atkins after a while on it because they never get into a state of ketosis.

Traditional keto is purposely a moderate-protein diet (around 20 to 25 percent of your calories) because you want to avoid giving your body too much glucose to run on, because then it will be bumped out of ketosis and you'll no longer be burning fat as fuel; you do this by limiting protein as well as carbs. At its heart keto is not so much about counting calories and avoiding certain foods for the sake of losing weight as it is about *biohacking your metabolism* so that your body functions optimally, and that means getting yourself into a state of ketosis. Just realize that protein thresholds will differ from person to person.

For me, keto isn't just about restricting your diet and losing weight; it's about turning your body into an optimally functioning machine so that you feel satiated, love what you're eating, lose weight, and gain all kinds of energy and mental clarity. So for me comparing it to Atkins is a bit of a dead end. Atkins will not get most people into a state of ketosis, and it certainly won't keep you there, and therefore the outcomes are more limited.

That said, I believe in customizing keto for every person. We're all different, and so getting you into a state of ketosis may be different from your spouse or neighbor or that shredded woman at the gym. Like I said, some bodybuilders can get into a state of ketosis on modified Atkins, but for most people, that balance of protein, fat, and carbohydrates won't have optimal effects. I'll give you some basic guidelines for getting into ketosis, but in phase two of my program, keto for the long term, I'll also teach you how to find out *your* protein and carbohydrate thresholds so that you can make keto work best for you.

MYTH #4:
Keto will cause muscle loss

People think high protein is what you need to produce muscle (if you've ever lived with a high school football player downing cases of high-protein Muscle Milk like it's their job, you'll know what I'm talking about). Therefore, the thinking goes, a lower-protein diet like keto must mean muscle loss.

Nope. In fact, ketones are very protein sparing. Your body will preserve its lean muscle mass in a state of ketosis and use fat as a primary source of fuel. Remember that ketones are a very efficient fuel source—the long-burning coals of the fire rather than the spikes and dips of lighter fluid (glucose).

I'll use myself as an example: I used to consume 180 to 200 grams of protein a day. Ever since I started on the ketogenic diet, I consume 80 to 120 grams of protein at the most. Over my two to three years on this diet, I've been able to maintain my muscle mass on half the amount of protein. I also

have more energy and mental clarity than I've ever had before. I don't like to brag about my rock-hard abs, so just believe me what I say: you will not lose muscle mass on the ketogenic diet unless you're eating at a calorie deficit over a long period of time, doing way too much cardio, and not lifting enough heavy things.

MYTH # 5:
It's not safe to do keto long-term

People often think of keto as a get-slim-fast diet that's only safe to do short-term, but that's a big misconception. It's a lifestyle change, and it's one that you can safely and easily incorporate into your life long-term. Remember those hunter-gatherer ancestors I talked about before? Spoiler alert: they weren't going into ketosis to trim inches off their waists. For them it was a normal and natural ebb and flow, and it can be that for us, too. In fact, the long-term benefits are the most common responses I get from people doing my program—I'm always hearing feedback like "I'm on a lifelong path that gives me more energy and a better life" or "What started as a 30-day diet has become a lifestyle. I'm in love with the way keto makes me feel and I'm going to stick with it for life."

It's true that for some time there wasn't much known about the long-term effects of keto because no one was studying it. Those days are gone. Today we know that the long-term effects of keto are much like the short-term: decreased inflammation, stellar weight management, decreased triglycerides, LDL cholesterol (the "bad" one), and blood glucose, and increased HDL cholesterol (the "good" one!).[7]

In Part 4 of this book I'll show you how to get the most out of keto long-term for your life and your health goals.

MYTH # 6
The ketogenic diet causes ketoacidosis

Ketoacidosis is a serious condition that typically happens in people with type 1 diabetes. You can die from it, so it's nothing to mess around with. In ketoacidosis, both ketone and glucose levels rise at the same time, to dangerous levels. The average person won't have this problem on the ketogenic diet because you produce enough insulin to moderate your ketone and glucose levels; when your ketone levels rise, your glucose drops and you experience no insulin spikes unless you kick yourself out of ketosis with a high-carb meal. But in a person with type 1 diabetes, your body lacks the ability to moderate those levels and they rise unchecked.

I always recommend that everyone on the ketogenic diet monitor their levels, and I'll talk more about how and why in the program section of this book. If you have type 1 diabetes, however, doing keto is a little bit tricky because of the extra and constant monitoring you'll have to do to make sure your levels of ketones and glucose are safe. If you have type 1 diabetes and you want to try a ketogenic diet, talk to your doctor first.

BONUS MYTH
YOU CAN'T DO KETO IF YOU DON'T HAVE A GALLBLADDER

I've had so many people message me asking if they can do keto without a gallbladder. Since it seems to be pretty common, I thought I'd address this common myth. The gallbladder helps process fat in the body. If you don't have one, it means you might have a harder time processing fat, but that doesn't mean you can't do keto; it means you'll want to start with a lower fat content to get started and find that threshold for yourself. I'd recommend starting with 50 percent fat and see how your body works on that. You may also want to take an ox bile supplement, which is a liver enzyme that will help you process fat.

BENEFITS OF A KETO LIFESTYLE

Now that we've got some of the most common myths out of the way, let's talk about some of my favorite *benefits* of keto. Bear with me here though; there are SO many benefits to keto and I want it to blow your mind the way it blew mine, so I'm going full speed ahead with all the latest info and research I could get my hands on. I'm betting by the end you'll feel exactly as I do— that KETO IS AMAZING!

The keto diet and lifestyle are becoming more and more studied, and it's all really good news, friend. Science shows positive outcomes for blood sugar management, mental focus, brain function, and so much more.

One of the first things most people notice when they start burning fat for fuel is that their cognitive function improves on the ketogenic diet. Many people feel more mental clarity and focus without the 3 P.M. crash and lethargy after a high-carb meal for lunch. This mental clarity becomes even more important as we age; the older we get, the more carb sensitive we become and the more our brain's ability to use glucose as an energy source is diminished over time. Increased energy, enhanced brain function, and better mental focus on keto are an outcome of increased blood flow to the brain. Keto can help reduce headaches and migraines, too.[8]

This is why the keto lifestyle is so popular with athletes, CEOs, celebrities, coaches, trainers, seven- to nine-figure entrepreneurs, and many other high performers—they are learning they can perform more optimally running off of ketones. They're utilizing the ketogenic diet to enhance their cognitive function and optimize their brain performance and YOU CAN TOO!!!

Improved cognitive function is the reason I fell in love with keto. Remember that movie *Limitless,* where Bradley Cooper's character takes these magical pills that allow him to use 100 percent of his brain and thus becomes a financial genius in minutes? It feels a little like that. I can't suddenly understand astrophysics or instantly pick up foreign languages, but I get through the day without needing to stop and eat and digest and get back to it—instead I'm going from recording my podcast to responding to emails to my workout to spending time with my daughters, and the whole time I feel great, like I'm running on jet fuel. If the foreign language thing happens, though, I'll be sure to let you know. Because that would be cool.

Research is also showing that keto offers some neuroprotective benefits in seizure disorders, can help treat ADHD, and may help prevent or slow down Alzheimer's disease by improving memory and cognitive function.[9] It's also been shown to improve the functioning of those with Parkinson's disease and multiple sclerosis.[10] Keto helps regulate brain chemicals to improve mood, too, making it a good support for anyone suffering from depression.[11]

I've already talked about how good keto is for your heart, and there's even more good news on that front. The ketogenic diet has been shown to improve triglyceride and cholesterol levels most associated with arterial buildup, and to increase HDL and decrease LDL particle concentration.[12] In fact, the most cutting-edge research shows that cholesterol levels alone are not good indicators of what causes heart attacks and that without carbs in the system, healthy fats can help prevent heart disease and stroke.[13]

As I said above, many of these benefits of the ketogenic diet all stem from its amazing anti-inflammatory abilities. You've probably heard that inflammation causes disease; the typical American diet is highly inflammatory, with high carbohydrate consumption, as well as high intake of processed foods and sugar-heavy foods. The ketogenic diet, on the other hand, is very anti-inflammatory, and this benefits all our body's systems. All that anti-inflammatory power is also crazy good for your skin; keto has been shown to support healing of acne and skin diseases.[14]

Keto has also been shown to regulate hormones—why? Because healthy fats are the building blocks of hormones. They are necessary for helping your body make the hormones it needs to function. And because fats surround cell walls and allow hormones to enter your cells, which helps them naturally balance.[15] On the other side of the coin, a low-fat diet has been linked to an imbalance of hormones. Any condition that arises from a hormonal imbalance, from polycystic ovary syndrome (PCOS) to fertility issues to endometriosis to low testosterone, can benefit from adding healthy fats into the diet. Hormones are communication systems in our bodies, and if one isn't working it's a snowball effect that can lead to a whole slew of issues for your body in the long run—so addressing your hormonal health will address the root causes of many other issues. For example, estrogen, progesterone, and testosterone are all steroid hormones made from cholesterol. So it would make sense that consumption of healthy saturated fats from things like coconut oil, MCT oil (which I'll talk about in Part 2), and fattier cuts of meat can help naturally increase these, whereas unhealthy fats like vegetable oil can lower them.

Researchers are also working on the theory that some cancers run on glucose and if you starve your body of glucose it can be good complementary care for cancer. Early research suggests that keto impedes the growth of cancerous tumors.[16] You read that right. There is so much amazing potential in the highly anti-inflammatory properties of keto.

And digestive and inflammation issues like gout and kidney stones? There's evidence that keto is good for those too. On keto you're not eating as often because you're not as hungry as often, giving your digestive system a break. In addition to this, many of the foods that cause digestive issues and inflammation are carbohydrates, so taking them out of the equation can be very restorative for gut health and digestive functioning.

Impressive, no? Mind = blown.

Studies have shown that keto can support blood sugar management and help lower levels of insulin, even for those with type 2 diabetes.[17] Keto's ability to help you manage your weight is extraordinary. As an appetite and craving suppressant, there's nothing else like it. The most up-to-date studies connect the keto diet and better performance at work, in the gym, and as a parent. It has been used for treating or managing everything from epilepsy to ADHD, and from depression to high cholesterol. The elimination of carbs has even been shown to improve acne.[18]

THE KETO MACROS

Getting your body into a state of ketosis so that you produce ketones and burn fat for fuel is the heart of the keto diet, and the keto macros are how you get there. With keto you don't necessarily need to count calories, you eat until you feel satiated. You do, however, watch your macros. "Macros" are your macronutrients, or the nutrients your body needs and consumes in large amounts: fats, carbs, and proteins. These are your "big" nutrients; your body converts these nutrients into energy, muscle, brain fuel, etc. All the big, important things that keep you alive. On keto, you're limiting carbohydrates and proteins and upping your fats so that your body goes into ketosis. When it comes to exact macronutrients on keto, there's so much bio-individuality (which is just a fancy way of saying "we're all different, y'all") that it's NOT a one-size-fits-all approach. But in general (meaning this will work for most people) on keto you should be getting approximately 75 percent of your calories from fat, 20 percent of your calories from protein, and 5 percent of your calories from carbohydrates each day.

The reason you're getting those in is that your main source of fuel is coming from fat. Too much protein or too much starch in the form of carbs will give your body glucose to run on, therefore preventing your backup system from kicking in and keeping you from being in a state of ketosis.

To give you a sense of what that might look like on an average day of keto, my CK30 meal plan, which was built with women in mind, is based on consuming approximately 1,500 calories per day. This breaks down to 125 grams fat, 75 grams protein, 19 grams carbs per day.

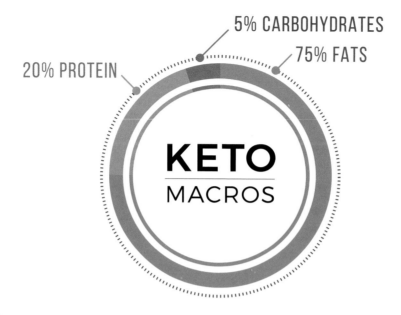

KETO MACROS

20% PROTEIN
5% CARBOHYDRATES
75% FATS

Men and some women may find they need to consume a little more, around 1,800 to 2,000 calories per day, and that breaks down to roughly 140 grams fat, 112 grams protein, 23 grams carbs per day. As I discuss in the Frequently Asked Questions section of Part 2, please don't consume less than 1,400 calories per day if you're a man and 1,100 calories per day if you're a woman. Remember: keto is not about counting calories or starving yourself— you want to eat and feel full. It's about limiting carbs and starches and upping your fats so that you get your body into a state of ketosis and burn fat for fuel.

Keep in mind that these macros are just a guideline—this will work to put most people in a state of ketosis, but you can't put everyone in a box. There's only one you! It's more important to get into ketosis than it is that you follow a guideline that isn't working for you.

For the first two weeks of the program I'll be asking you to track your macros and test to see if you're in ketosis. (I'll discuss how to do this in Part 2, and in Part 4 I'll discuss how to adjust your macros for doing keto long-term.) After those two weeks of tracking and testing you'll know if your body is in ketosis, so from there on out I encourage you to stop all the information gathering so you're not obsessing over your numbers. I want you to track where you are only in the beginning, so you have a baseline, and then stop so you don't get caught up in trying to be perfect. Instead, my goal is to help you to listen to your body and begin to start eating intuitively. Only eat when you are hungry and then stop when you are satisfied. I know it sounds simple, and I know it's not easy for everyone. It is possible, though. I promise. And I know you can do hard things.

"Macros" are talked about a lot when it comes to keto, but my program also includes lots of "micros"—micronutrients—as well. Micronutrients are things like vitamins, minerals, and phytonutrients. While macronutrients

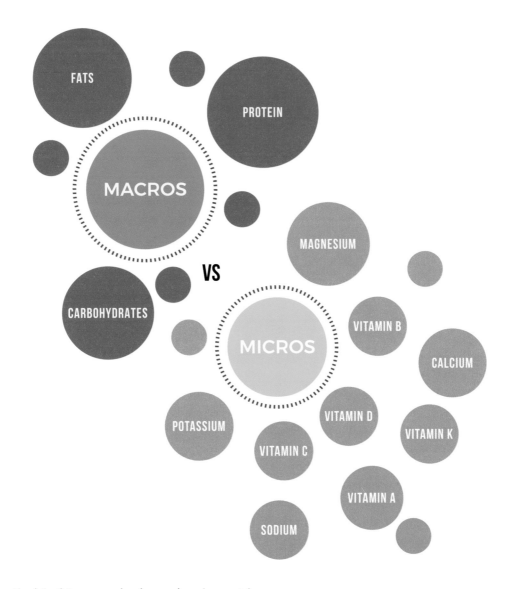

are the big things your body needs, micronutrients are the things you need to not just survive but thrive. It's not just about fats and carbs; you need vitamins and minerals, too. You'll see that my recipes include leafy greens and nutrient-dense non-starchy vegetables that are full of micronutrients and not a lot of carbs. This will keep you healthy and optimal.

VEGAN AND VEGETARIAN KETO MACROS

When doing veg*n keto, it can be more difficult to find foods to eat because you can't eat foods like eggs, meat, dairy, and fish. Therefore, my veg*n keto recommendation is that instead of counting total carbs to come

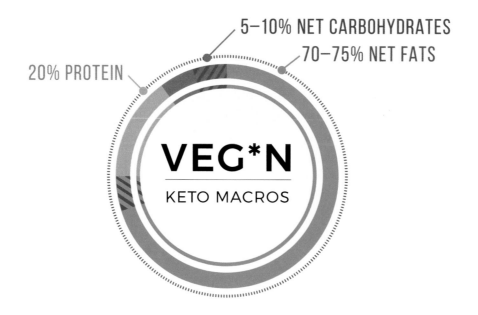

20% PROTEIN

5–10% NET CARBOHYDRATES

70–75% NET FATS

VEG*N
KETO MACROS

up with your daily macros, you'll count net carbs. While your fat and protein intake will stay the same as the omnivore plan, you'll be able to consume an average of 20 to 40 grams of *net carbs* per day, rather than the stricter 19 grams of total carbs on my omnivore plan. Total carbs are simply the total grams of carbs in your food. Net carbs are total carbs minus grams of fiber; we can discount the fiber because it doesn't cause the same blood sugar spike as other forms of carbs. Sometimes certain net carbs will kick people out of ketosis, but for you that matters less to me than that you're eating filling, satiating meals and not feeling hungry. I want you have more wiggle room when it comes to carbohydrates so that you are getting enough to eat. Like the omnivore plan, my veg*n meal plan is based on consuming approximately 1,500 calories per day, and for you this breaks down to 125 grams fat (70 to 75 percent of your total calories), 75 grams protein (approximately 20

percent of your total calories), and 20 to 40 grams net carbs per day (5 to 10 percent of your total calories). This will enable you to get more nutrients from vegetables.

WHAT TO EAT ON A KETO DIET

Okay, okay, keto is great for me, you are probably saying, but what can I actually eat, Drew?

When people think of limiting carbs, they often think of cutting out bread and pasta, but there are other foods that are high in carbs—including fruit, beans, rice, and some starchy veggies. You'll notice that the following lists of what to eat and what to avoid on keto break things like veggies and fruits down by high starch/carb and low or no starch/carb. I think you'll be pretty amazed by what you'll be eating, too. Let's take a look:

ANIMAL PROTEINS

BEEF	BISON	POULTRY
VEAL	LAMB	EGGS
	PORK	

Grass-fed, organic, hormone free, antibiotic free, and free range are best options if your budget allows. Remember, lean cuts of meat are okay, but increase fat from other sources when enjoying them.

SEAFOOD

CATFISH	SNAPPER	SHELLFISH
COD	TROUT	LOBSTER
FLOUNDER	TUNA	CRAB
HALIBUT	SARDINES	MUSSELS
MACKEREL	(preferably in olive oil)	SQUID
MAHI MAHI	OYSTERS	TUNA
SALMON	CLAMS	SHRIMP

Wild-caught is a better option than farmed if your budget allows. Remember, lean cuts of fish are okay, but increase fat from other sources when enjoying them.

FATS & OILS

OLIVE OIL	AVOCADO OIL	PALEO MAYONNAISE
COCONUT OIL	GHEE	MACADAMIA OIL
MCT OIL	LARD	

Grass-fed and organic sources of these are best options if your budget allows.

VEGETABLES

ASPARAGUS	CHILI PEPPERS	PICKLES
ARUGULA	COLLARD GREENS	OLIVES
BELL PEPPERS (LIMITED)	CUCUMBERS	ONIONS (LIMITED)
BOK CHOY	GARLIC	PUMPKIN
BROCCOLI	GINGER ROOT	RADISHES
BROCCOLINI	GREEN BEANS	ROMAINE LETTUCE
BRUSSEL SPROUTS	GREEN ONIONS	SAUERKRAUT
BUTTER LEAF LETTUCE	HERBS	SPAGHETTI SQUASH
CABBAGE	ICEBERG LETTUCE	SPINACH
CAULIFLOWER	KALE	TURNIPS
CELERY	KIMCHI	YELLOW SQUASH
CHARD	MUSHROOMS	ZUCCHINI

LIQUIDS

COFFEE	WATER	SPARKLING WATER
TEA		(plain or naturally flavored like La Croix, Perrier, and Zevia)

FRUITS

AVOCADO	BLUEBERRIES	BLACKBERRIES
TOMATOES	STRAWBERRIES	RASPBERRIES

Consume fruits in very limited quantities,
as these do have higher carbs.

DAIRY/NUTS/SEEDS

BUTTER	MACADAMIA NUTS	PUMPKIN SEEDS
HEAVY CREAM	CASHEWS	SUNFLOWER SEEDS
CHEESE	PECANS	CHIA SEEDS
SOUR CREAM	WALNUTS	FLAXSEEDS
CREAM CHEESE	ALMONDS	NATURAL NUT BUTTER

As you'll see in Part 3, I don't include dairy, nuts, or seeds on my CK30 plan, but if you choose to enjoy them, do so in limited quantities as these are inflammatory and can easily be overconsumed. Nuts also have some carbs, so you must take them into consideration for your daily total. This list is also helpful if you decide to do keto long-term and want to bring dairy, nuts, and seeds back in after the first 30 days.

Okay, so you can have bacon (unless you're vegetarian or vegan, in which case, don't worry, I've got recipes, tips, and support for you, too!). I've got you covered with lots of recipes and meal ideas in the program section. But maybe at this point you're already starting to wonder what an average day of keto looks like? Well, here's a sample to give you an idea:

➤ Meal 1 around 7 A.M.: Drew's Keto Coffee

➤ Meal 2 around noon: Chicken cobb salad, no croutons, no cheese, with avocado and olive oil mixed with vinegar and mustard for dressing.

➤ Meal 3 around 6 P.M.: 6-ounce rib eye steak topped with ghee and broccoli, sautéed in avocado oil, on the side.

WHAT TO AVOID ON A KETO DIET

Take a look at the graphic on page 20 for a visual reminder of what not to eat if you're eating keto! Stay away from starchy veggies (potatoes, sweet potatoes, carrots, etc.), fruits (except for very limited amounts), grains, chips, cookies, crackers, rice, pasta, cereals, juices, and sodas.

Note to my veg*n friends: Does that list of meat and fish freak you out? Don't worry, you too can do keto. I've got you covered with a sample veg*n meal plan in the program and lots of delicious recipes that will keep you on your game *and* give you all the benefits of keto.

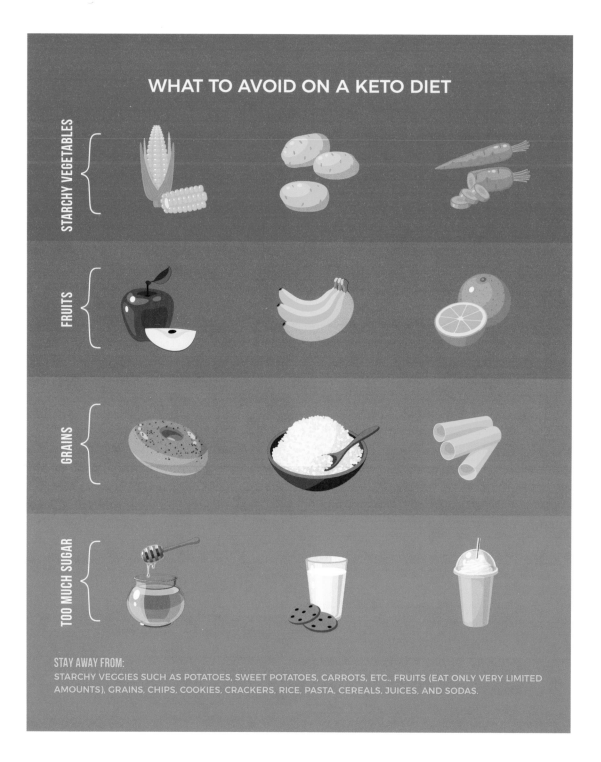

WHAT TO AVOID ON A KETO DIET

STARCHY VEGETABLES

FRUITS

GRAINS

TOO MUCH SUGAR

STAY AWAY FROM:
STARCHY VEGGIES SUCH AS POTATOES, SWEET POTATOES, CARROTS, ETC., FRUITS (EAT ONLY VERY LIMITED AMOUNTS), GRAINS, CHIPS, COOKIES, CRACKERS, RICE, PASTA, CEREALS, JUICES, AND SODAS.

WHAT TO EAT FOR VEG*NS

PROTEIN

TOFU

TEMPEH TVP

LOW-CARB PROTEIN POWDER

BAKING

ALMOND FLOUR/MEALS

COCONUT FLOUR

FLAXSEED MEAL

PSYLLIUM HUSK

ANY UNSWEETENED NONDAIRY MILK

FATS & OILS

COCONUT OIL

MCT OIL

ALMOND BUTTER

VEGETABLES

Same as omnivore list, but with some additional veggies,
'cause I know how my veg*ns roll.

ARTICHOKES
ASPARAGUS
AVOCADO
BOK CHOY
BRUSSELS SPROUTS
CABBAGE

NUTS & SEEDS

ALMONDS
CASHEWS
CHIA SEEDS
COCONUT FLAKES
HAZELNUTS

FRUITS & LIQUIDS

Same as omnivore plan

If you're already wondering what a day of veg*n keto might look like, here's a sample:

➤ Meal 1 around 7 A.M.: Chocolate Peanut Butter Shake

➤ Meal 2 around noon: Greek Salad

➤ Meal 3 around 6 P.M.: Broccoli Stir Fry

➤ Snack: ½ cup whole almonds + ¼ cup sunflower seeds

WHAT DO I DO IF I HATE AVOCADOS?

Um, learn to love them? Just kidding. I get questions like this a lot. What to do on keto if you hate avocados, coconut, etc. It's easy. Simply replace avocado (or whatever it is you don't like) with any other approved fat from the food list. I like adding avocado or olive oil to really up the fats. But you can do whatever you enjoy and stands out to you.

WOMEN ON KETO

If you're a keto-curious woman who is unsure if the lifestyle is for you because you associate keto with ripped men doing CrossFit—let me take a minute right here to say that it's not an all-boys club by any means. A lot of bio-individuality goes into this diet and lifestyle. It's not a magic pill or a one-size-fits-all program.

Keto is not about intimidating gym scenes: it's a lifestyle that gives you energy, makes you love your body, and enables you to take control of your health. There are no gender prerequisites for that.

There is some evidence that eliminating carbohydrates as you do in the ketogenic lifestyle helps regulate women's hormones and lowers their testosterone—and, since the culprit of conditions like PCOS is often elevated testosterone, keto potentially reduces the effects of PCOS.[19] Women with high testosterone tend to do very well on keto because this is often a sign of other imbalances—like insulin resistance, estrogen or progesterone imbalances, high DHEA, or high liptins. Since all these hormones are connected like a web, when you regulate one you begin to regulate the others. The hormone regulation you get from keto may even help with fertility.[20]

That said, if you're trying to get pregnant—or if you're pregnant or nursing—I wouldn't suggest trying something new now. If you want to consider going keto, be sure to talk with your medical provider first.

If you're a woman reading this, can I talk to you over here for a minute? Shhh, don't tell the men reading this book, but as you'll see in Parts 3 and 4, my program is actually designed with you in mind. Any modifications for men are given as notes to the program, usually just some information about increasing portions.

Women are too often left out in health and weight loss programs or given an afterthought status, which doesn't really make a lot of sense to me, especially when I read that this secondary status actually hurts women's health when it comes to things like heart attack and stroke. It felt like the least I could do to put you first in this book. Now back to our regularly scheduled programming.

EMOTIONAL SUPPORT FOR YOUR JOURNEY

So now you know what keto is. We've dispelled some of the biggest myths about keto and you know all the many benefits of keto. You have a sense of the foods to eat and avoid. Hopefully you're feeling excited and motivated to try this new lifestyle! But wait—how exactly do you tackle those mental and emotional struggles that have prevented you from starting or continuing a lifestyle change in the past? Don't worry, I got you covered.

My tried-and-true hacks for overcoming emotional challenges with food will flow throughout this whole book. Here let me start by giving you five things you can do for emotional support on your keto journey:

1. Find your why

What's the reason you're doing all this? Why are you getting healthy and taking care of yourself? What do you want all that mental clarity for? Your answer(s) to these questions is what I call your "why"—and naming it is important for motivating you through those hard times when you just want to give up.

It has to be more than wanting to look good or be skinny—there's got to be a bigger why than that. I know that looking good and losing weight may be your primary reasons for picking up this book and doing keto, and I know those aren't small things; they're powerful and meaningful. But it can't stop there, because being skinny or looking great in your jeans or impressing everyone at your high school reunion are all cool things, but they're not going to motivate you for the rest of your life. Same with things like money and fame. Those things are fine, but you need something bigger than yourself and your looks to believe in to truly motivate you in the long term.

Think deep about what brings you fulfillment in life. Now you might be saying, well, eating donuts makes me feel good, and believe me, I know that feeling, but I wouldn't say eating donuts is fulfilling—I wouldn't say it's a why any more than I'd say fame or thinness is a why. A why is about something bigger: think relationships, family, friends, memories, passion, purpose, and finding your joy and meaning in life.

For me, one of my whys is being a dad. Having my daughters, being an example to them, being able to give them the best life I can possibly give them, making memories with them, having experiences with them—this all gives my life meaning and gives me reason to keep pushing myself to meet my goals. My other big why is helping people transform: hearing your stories, hearing you overcome hardships and do the impossible—that kind of stuff fulfills my soul to the core.

So what brings you fulfillment? Sit back and think about it for as long as you need to. When you come up with an answer, write it down. Now you've got your why. As you move forward on this keto journey, keep your why with you—maybe write it down and keep it in your pocket or near your bed or desk. Whenever you feel overwhelmed or wanting to give up, remember your why, and it will help you keep going.

2. Publicly announce your goals

Post on social media. Talk to friends and family. Tell people what your intentions are. Be as specific as you can be: What do you hope to achieve with keto? Why are you doing keto? What's your plan? What program are you doing?

Announcing your intentions or goals to the masses can be scary for sure. What if I fail? What if I look dumb? What if I can't do it? All these doubts go through our minds.

I once spoke with this amazingly kind dude named Brian. He was married but felt that being obese and not very active was pushing this woman he loved away. So after some research, he found my program and decided to do keto for her. He shared this plan with her and was really stoked to get started. Two months in he was feeling great and was down 30 pounds. Then his wife left him. He was devastated. He thought about quitting. But then he decided, you know what? I owe this to *myself*. Lightbulb! New intention. He

joined a gym and signed up for some workout classes. He eventually signed up for his first 5K. Today he's still going strong and planning even more challenges and adventures with all the energy he's found. His new friends at the gym and in class are the people he announces every new goal to these days. And they couldn't be happier for him.

It's hard to put yourself out there for someone—and it's maybe even harder to put yourself out there for you. But you have to know why you're making this lifestyle change. You have to be willing to be really honest with yourself about it if you want to stay motivated. And you have to be willing to tell others, even knowing they might not get it. That's just an opportunity to figure out your new intention—maybe a deeper, more rewarding intention in the end.

During my journey back to fit in my Fit2Fat2Fit journey, I had so many cravings and temptations where I wanted to give in sometimes. Every time I walked past the aisle with Cinnamon Toast Crunch or I'd see a Mountain Dew ad (have you ever noticed that they're *everywhere*?!), it brought back those feelings—those cravings. And I mean strong cravings—like the ones where you can still taste the soft crunch and the hit of those sugar crystals hitting your tongue, where you can still smell the aroma when you first opened the box and you knew the way it made you feel. It made your brain light up like the Fourth of July of pure excitement and joy because this food tasted so damn good. I'd think, "no one will notice if I just have one," or "nobody will see me guzzling the Dew in my car, so why not?" And then someone would walk down the cereal aisle and I'd remember how I posted my plan so publicly. What if someone did see me? What if they said, "Hey aren't you that Fit2Fat2Fit guy? Aren't you on your journey back to Fit now? Why are you eating Cinnamon Toast Crunch?" That fear of getting caught kept me from giving in to my temptations.

More than that, though, knowing that there were people doing this journey with me (literally thousands of people—strangers, friends, people who were depending on me) made me think, if they're doing it I can do it, too. The power of accountability is huge and way too underestimated, IMHO.

3. Find a support system

You don't just need to make your intentions public; you also need a strong support team in place to carry you through the ups and downs. Who's excited about your goals and dreams? Who's on your team?

Maybe it's your family and friends—or maybe it's not. We often think our loved ones will be supportive, but they can sabotage us too. It's not because they don't love you; it's probably because they're afraid: of change, of losing you, of losing the things they love to do with you. So if you find that family and friends aren't the support system you need, try to keep in mind where they're coming from, send a big dose of forgiveness and grace their way, and find your support elsewhere.

Maybe it's a Facebook community (like mine, Complete Keto Book, which I'd love for you to join) or an app. Maybe it's a coach or personal trainer. There are seemingly endless ways to connect with people these days—reach out and find some good people to help you stay accountable to yourself and your goals.

Remember that final scene in the movie *Rudy*? You know the one—where you're definitely not crying but there's something in your eye that you need a tissue for or you're just sweating from your eyeballs? The moment when this guy who dreamed of playing Notre Dame football and all the odds are stacked against him—he's homeless, can't afford college, doesn't have good enough grades to get in anyway, and isn't exactly the most athletic dude—miraculously is on the team and gets called in to the game? And the whole, absolutely jam-packed, stadium starts chanting "Rudy! Rudy! Rudy!" And then he sacks the quarterback and gets carried off the field on his teammates' shoulders in full glory? Yeah. *That's* how your support system should make you feel. Be the Rudy of your own movie. Find those people who'll wholeheartedly chant for you on your journey to overcome all your own obstacles. And while you're at it, be the one cheering your head off for others who are doing the same.

Don't forget the community you have because you're reading this book—be sure to visit our Facebook group, like I said above, and check out all the bonus material you can download at my website, fit2fat2fit.com /completeketobook.

4. Stay accountable

If you're like me, you like to follow people in the fitness industry who've inspired you—and at times I've got a handful of people in my social media feeds who used to be on shows like *The Biggest Loser*, *Extreme Weight Loss*, or my show, *Fit to Fat to Fit*, and others. 'Cause I'm rooting for them. But I can always tell when they've taken a downhill turn in their journey because the show ends, and a once-busy social media account goes inactive. I know this likely means they've starting gaining weight back, they feel ashamed, and they don't want to talk about it. The commonality among those people who are the most successful? They stay active on these accounts. I'm not saying they are all perfect all the time. I'm saying they show you their journey—their struggles, successes, failures, all of it. They keep posting.

Take Ali Vincent, for example. Ali was the first woman to win *The Biggest Loser*. A few years after appearing on the show, Ali found herself weighing close to her weight before the show. She felt ashamed, embarrassed, and overwhelmed. But she didn't just disappear when she struggled. Instead Ali went public, announcing her fears and her plan on her Facebook page. She shared that she was joining Weight Watchers and that she had decided to be done with shame. "I remember wondering before if I was unhappy because I was heavy or heavy because I was unhappy, I realized it didn't matter because both were true and I needed to do something about it," Ali

wrote. "I've decided to feel proud of myself again! To hell with shame! I've been so afraid and worried of public shame and ridicule that I've created more pain for myself than anyone else can but not anymore." Ali kept posting, and kept herself accountable to her followers. In doing so she gave us a gift better than the inspiration of achieving her weight loss goal: she gave us her vulnerability and her honesty. She helps us see that we're all in this thing together, that we all struggle, and that we can empower each other to keep going when the going gets tough. No shame, only love.

Create your own version of this accountability. Whether it's a social media account, a blog, a vlog, or a journal you keep. Making your goals public is important, but that won't do anything for you if it's a one-and-done thing. Stay accountable. Keep putting yourself out there, even when the going is tough—especially when the going is tough! Talk about your journey. Talk about your challenges. Talk about the goals you meet and the ones you don't. All of that—just keep posting about it, whether you have one follower or 1,000.

I encourage you to continually put yourself outside your comfort zone—sign up for a 5K, triathlon, Spartan race, Tough Mudder, Ragnar race, physique competition, or some other kind of competition—especially if you have to put money down on it. When you commit those dollar bills it gives you a whole other level of investment. You can even join something like dietbet.com where you put money into a pot and bet on yourself. If you bet money on yourself, you're so much more likely to achieve your goals. Or maybe try the opposite approach—there are sites out there where you can bet money on yourself and if you don't meet your goal that money gets donated to an organization you hate.

Why does this work? Because as I said above, you need to have a bigger *why*. You need something that's bigger than you. Then you can focus on keeping going rather than perfection. Focus on being open and honest with yourself and your support team rather than keeping your macros perfect and your weight loss on schedule.

5. Ditch the scale

Get rid of it. For real.

Imagine you're looking in the mirror and you're totally naked and you see *your* perfect body. You look amazing. You love the way your body looks. You're really feeling yourself. Would you care at all how much you weighed?

Or imagine you're looking in the mirror totally naked and you see yourself in *your* perfect health—aches and pains gone, fatigue gone, no more bloating, strong and confident. Would it matter how much you weighed?

Look, I understand the appeal of the scale—weight is an easy way to measure change. But the problem with weighing yourself is that we let our weight define us. It just doesn't really mean that much. It's our relationship to gravity, people. Why do

we as humans put so much value on our relationship with gravity? It's silly, really, if you think about it. Our weight is constantly changing throughout the day. Yet we give it so much power over us, this inconsistent thing. We let that number define us—and even worse, we let it control our emotions. When the number on the scale is going down we're happy, excited, and proud. When it's going up we feel frustrated and stressed, anxious and disappointed. We can let it get us so stressed that we're missing the benefits of the lifestyle change.

I caught this story once a few years back—January Harshe, a mother of six and founder of Birth Without Fear, agreed to get photos of herself taken at her highest weight in *nothing but her underwear* for something called the 4th Trimester Bodies Project. Which means these photos would be posted on the Internet. To her half-million followers and whoever else came across them. Her message? Her reason for doing this? "Loving yourself to health is not the same as hating yourself to skinny." That is some real talk right there.

It's not that this woman didn't struggle with loving her body—she did. It's not that she didn't have her own weight loss and health goals—she did. But she was brave enough to put all her vulnerabilities and body image issues out there for the whole world to see to share the message that it's really all about the journey, not the destination (isn't that a Miley Cyrus song?).

If I could bottle this badass mama's vibe to give you, I would. Because what

HOW TO TAKE MEASUREMENTS OF YOUR BODY

A. CHEST
B. WAIST
C. HIPS

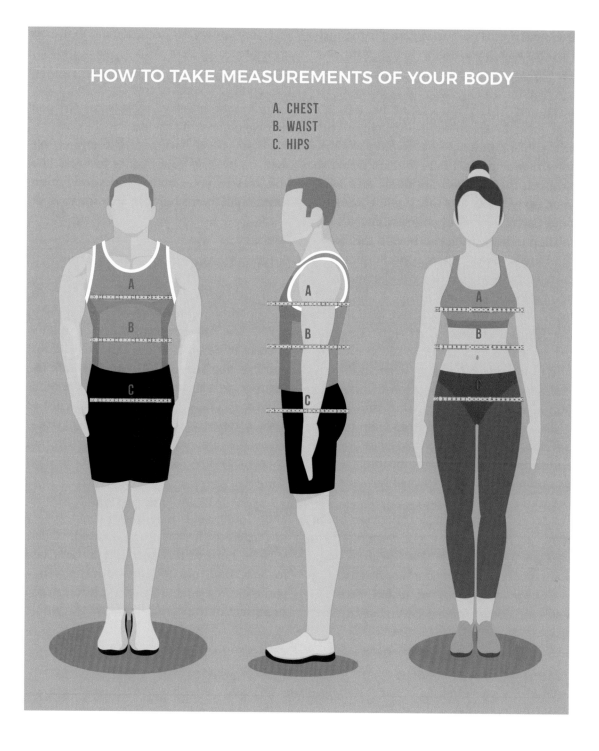

true health is, is not just *results*. It's the process. It's loving yourself to health. And *your* healthy on *your* body looks different than *my* healthy on *my* body and every other Instagram fitness model's body, too. It's practicing being mindful and happy with who you are right now while you're working toward your goals. I believe it's possible to love you for who you are today and what your body looks like today while working on a better version of yourself, and it's my mission to help teach you how in this book.

Here's a secret: there is no finish line. A certain number on a scale won't actually tell you that much about yourself, and it won't fix everything for you. We have long lives to live; let's not waste them striving for a number on a scale. You have so much more to offer this world other than what your body looks like. Let's make peace with ourselves now *and* rock our weight loss and health goals. I want keto to help you learn how to develop a better relationship with yourself and focus on the process, not the results. I want to help you love yourself now and put progress over perfection.

So get rid of the scale. There are better forms of measurement. For example, take measurements with a tape measure: your waist, your chest, and your hips at least.

Or get your body fat tested instead— ask your doctor for a DEXA scan or BOD POD assessment, or just google one in your area. Stay consistent with it; get a baseline of whatever form of measurement you can use, and every week or two weeks, or at least every month, check your progress. The goal isn't weight loss, it's fat loss.

If you don't have access to any of this, then go by how your clothes feel and how you feel in your body. That's way more meaningful than a number on a scale.

6. Don't compare yourself to others

I believe it was Roosevelt who said, "Comparison is the thief of joy." Hashtag truth. See, the problem with comparing yourself to others is that it can mean almost nothing. You may say, "I want to look like that person," and that makes you feel motivated for a while, but then you could just as easily compare yourself to someone in worse shape than you are and then say, "Oh, no, I'm actually doing fine," and your motivation is gone.

It's like you go to your neighbor's house and it's immaculate. Perfectly clean, totally uncluttered, brilliantly decorated. Okay, let's be honest, this probably annoys you for a second, but then it motivates you— you make it a goal to finally go through the basement or the garage and give the whole house a deep cleaning. Say then you go to another friend's house the next day and this home is cluttered and in disarray. Dog hair everywhere. Toys strewn all over the place. Dishes in the sink. Maybe the faint smell of something no longer ripe in the fruit bowl. And you think, well, my house is spotless compared to this! There goes your motivation. When you hang your motivation on comparison to others, you can always find someone doing "better" than you and someone doing "worse"—in the end, comparison is a flimsy source of inspiration because it's external validation and that can change from day to day, minute to minute.

The real questions are: what are *your* unique, individual goals and what is *your* why? There is no one perfect outcome—it's so individualized. Consider these testimonials from three different women:

"I've not lost a single pound on keto but I've gained more muscle mass and strength than I'd ever thought possible, and I can fit in clothes that I thought were destined for the thrift store."

"I've lost 58 pounds in 6 months!"

"I stopped weighing myself a while back so I don't know how much I've lost, and honestly I don't care. All I know is I feel great, my clothes fit great, and I have more energy than I ever had before. I went to see my doctor recently and he can't believe that I've reversed my hypertension diagnosis and that all my labs came back in the normal range."

Here are three stories of improved health, and yet they look very different. One woman didn't lose any weight—and in fact gained more mass—but fits in her clothes better; one woman lost almost 60 pounds; and the third woman doesn't even weigh herself, but charts her progress by her energy and her lab work. I have hundreds more stories like these! Believe me when I say that there is no one perfect outcome.

The problem is that we see Instagram models and we think that's what health is—that's what it should look like to be healthy. The truth is that healthy looks different on everybody.

When we say we want to look just like someone else, we are equating physical transformation with happiness. But you are not that other person and losing 20 pounds will not magically fix everything in your life. That person is not you and will never be you, nor would you want them to be, honestly. Physical transformation does not equate to happiness. It has to come from within. You create your own happiness. You can only compete with you. Are you a better person than you were yesterday? Six months ago? A year ago? That's your competition. No one else. Mic drop.

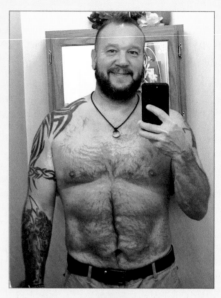

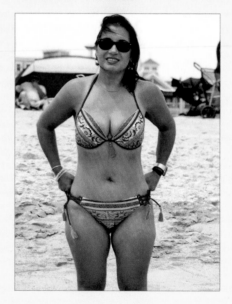

BEFORE

AFTER

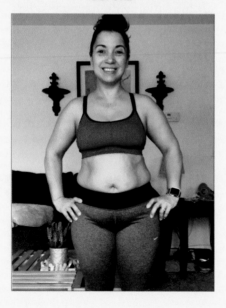

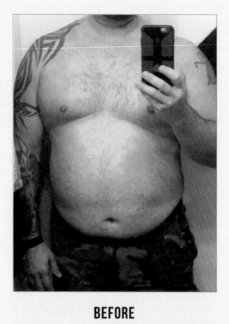

JOSH & MIRIAM MARTIN

I STARTED MY WEIGHT LOSS JOURNEY/CHALLENGE A FEW YEARS BACK WHEN I weighed in at 340 pounds. I'd lose and gain and lose and gain until I was so frustrated I didn't care. I justified it by telling myself that my career as a corrections officer required me to be bigger. Unfortunately it made me a slower, lazier officer who was very ineffective after what would be a short jog for most (an all-out run for me), thus putting my fellow officers in jeopardy. This, of course, ran over into my home life, where bigger also isn't better. I was also a slower, lazier husband to a beautiful wife and father to adorable twin girls. Girls who love to run, play, chase butterflies, etc. . . . Not me, though.

Feeling pretty down about it, I came across this video of a very "robust" dude chasing his little one around his kitchen seemingly very winded. I could relate. I could relate 100 percent. I'm sure you all know the Drew Manning video I'm talking about. I looked him up and saw what it was all about. I couldn't believe this guy went from being in incredible shape to trying to be a "fat guy" like me. ON PURPOSE! I was a little offended until I saw the other side of his accomplishment. It was then I said, "Why not me?" I was in decent shape at one time—not recently, but for a while. I was a gym rat for years.

I decided to start my new "crazy keto" way of eating because it was pretty much the only thing I hadn't tried. I started the day after my Patriots lost the Super Bowl. I calculated my macros and food prepped and was ready to roll. As of this morning I've lost just over 50 pounds (99 total) and weighed in at 241. A number I have not seen since my early 20s. I started at three meals a day, working down to one meal a day. I make sure to hit my macros accordingly and drop them as my weight decreases.

I've completely reversed my fatty liver, and as of my last appointment, according to my doctor, I have the kidney function of a teenager. 179 cholesterol, down from 360. 125/80 BP, from 165/110 (borderline stroke victim, so he said). This is the first time since I've met this guy that as I walked out he told me I looked great. Obviously till that day I didn't.

I have to say that I could not have done this without my amazingly beautiful wife, Miriam. She has supported me the entire way. She also began her keto journey around that same time, roughly three weeks later. She has accomplished goals that were previously thought to be unattainable. She's killing it! We are never going back to our old selves. Never!

I also gotta give props to the guy who wanted to know what it felt like to be me. I'm gonna do my best to return the favor. My wife, little girls, and co-workers: thank you as well. They all finally have the man who's always gonna be there whether they need me or not.

— JOSH MARTIN

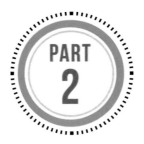

PART 2

GETTING STARTED

Now that you know what keto is, how and why it works, the many benefits of keto, and the basics of what to eat and what to avoid, you're ready to look at how to get started on the journey. Whether you're a health and fitness pro or you've never followed a diet plan in your life, this section will hold your hand and walk you through everything you need to know to jump into my CK30 plan with confidence in Part 3. No matter your background, I'm so happy you're here now, in this space of no judgment, no shame, only love and empathy, getting ready to embark on this journey.

I know from my own journey that getting started and sticking with it is as much about the mental and emotional aspects as it is about the physical. I could give you the best meal plans ever, with the healthiest, cleanest sources of food and the perfect macros for you, and the best workout program, with top-of-line gym equipment recommendations and the perfect trainer for you, but *none* of that matters unless you figure out how to name and conquer your own demons. So before I get into the specific details, testing, travel, side effects, and more, I want to talk a little bit about one of the biggest emotional obstacles I've seen people get stuck on: putting pressure on ourselves.

My friend Amy was one of those "I've tried everything and nothing has worked" people. She shared with my Facebook group that she'd spent her adult life trying pretty much every diet: Atkins, paleo, Weight Watchers, SlimFast, and Jenny Craig, not to mention workouts like CrossFit, bootcamps, yoga, and working with a personal trainer at her gym. Nothing, she said, got her the results she was looking for. I could tell she was frustrated and overwhelmed, yet determined. She said her doctor had been warning her about her high cholesterol and high blood pressure for years and she was committed to making a change. She joined my Facebook group and signed up for my 30-day Keto Jumpstart program because she wanted to be there when her granddaughter was born, she shared with us, and to watch her grow.

She started the first week really strong, sharing her why with the group and some "before" photos. But then she reported back that she fell off the wagon. So she started again, only to share at the end of the week that she'd given up once more. Start and stop, start and stop. What's that definition of insanity? Doing the same thing over and over again and expecting different results. Something was not working.

I wanted to help her succeed so I commented on one of her posts, asking her about her relationship with the food on the plan. What foods were the hardest for her to give up? Which were the hardest to add? "I really like the foods in the beginning," she said. "I feel totally committed. I'm ready to change everything in my life and be a new me. But then I start craving bad things like cake and ice cream. If I let myself have a bite of cake I start hating myself, and then I just give up completely. Because I've already failed, I might as well not try."

It was a big aha! moment for me in terms of what was going on for Amy. I'd been there before on my Fit2Fat2Fit journey and heard similar stories from so many other people over the years. Amy's problem wasn't the food, or the meal prep, or her determination; it was that she was putting so much pressure on herself to be perfect. She was treating this diet like a religion she had to follow, and when she "failed" to follow it, she punished herself with negative self-talk and gave up.

So often we try to make things black-and-white—especially when it comes to dieting—that we end up getting dogmatic about what we are and aren't eating. Lots of people end up looking at their diet as a religion you have to follow or you'll be unhealthy or you'll die. It's easy for so many of us to get fixated on "Oh, this is not keto, this is keto," and from there we can start looking at keto foods and ingredients as good and anything that's not as evil, bad, or sinful things.

Even worse, this way of thinking can lead us to believe that the people who consume those "bad" foods that are not keto-approved are also bad or less than—including ourselves. It can lead us to feel that we're better than the people we love just because they're eating bread or a cupcake, or that we aren't good enough if we can't stop craving sweets or chips. I admit I used to feel this way before my Fit2Fat2Fit journey. I looked at people who couldn't say no to ice cream and sugary cereal as weak and lacking in willpower. I put that pressure on myself too. I had to be perfect all the time. I've seen others take this thinking even further—becoming so extreme they make people feel shame or guilt if they drink a beer or eat a banana.

As I travel the world bringing the keto lifestyle to people, they will often make a big deal if they see me enjoying a glass of wine, eating dessert, or even having a handful of blueberries. But you know what? I'm a human being. Yes, I live keto as a full-time lifestyle, but I also like to indulge every now and then. I keep it in context: If I enjoy something today, what does that mean for my macros? What will that mean for how I'll eat tomorrow? I get to choose. It doesn't have to be do-or-die. I don't want keto to become a religion for you. I don't want you to feel so chained to your macros app that you miss a great dinner with your family, like you're worshipping at the altar of the almighty scale or looking down on your own kids for wanting cake on their birthday. It's not about perfection. It's about loving the journey. Forgive yourself. Enjoy yourself. Give yourself the space you need to enjoy the ride.

I shared my philosophy with Amy, and she said she totally identified with putting this amount of pressure on herself and was ecstatic to hear someone finally say "enough." Other members of the group chimed in with their stories of ups and downs, and learning to love the process. A few weeks later she shared her "after." She had stuck with it. Did she mess up sometimes? Absolutely. But she kept going. A few months later she'd lost 50 pounds, and her doctor was blown away by her blood pressure and the cholesterol levels. Just as important, she told me she now has

more energy, is having more fun than ever before, and can't wait to run around playing with her granddaughter. All because she gave herself permission to be present to her life and to give up the illusion of perfection.

As you read the following pages in preparation for getting started on keto, keep Amy's story in mind and understand that all the guidelines and tips I offer are meant to support you, not judge or shame you. It's information to help make your experience better, not hard-and-fast rules. If you can start your journey by giving yourself lots of space to change and grow, and lots of self-love, I promise you'll be more likely to enjoy the ride, especially when things get tough.

KEEP IT IN CONTEXT: THE ANTIDOTE TO STRIVING FOR PERFECTION

When it comes to keto as a lifestyle, rather than thinking about things in black and white, think about keeping it all in context. Can you have cake and bread on keto? Maybe a bite, sure. But think of it this way: it's not the smartest use of your carbs for your body, because there go all your carbs for the day and you haven't gotten any micronutrients from that slice of bread or piece of cake. On the other hand, you can have a whopping 30 grams of nutrient-dense food like broccoli, kale, or Brussels sprouts or other non-starchy vegetables—things that do a lot of good for your body. If you want to have something with sucralose or alcohol, you can justify drinking it every once in a while, but you don't want to live on that stuff because it's not offering your body or your brain very much. It's not that some foods are "good" and some are "bad"—it's that some give you more bang for your buck. Some are chock-full of phytonutrients, vitamins, minerals, good healthy fats, protein, et cetera, and some are mostly just empty calories. Don't think of it as a piece of cake that's "bad" for you—think of it in the big-picture context of your life.

I'm not saying this as a fitness expert; I'm saying this as an average guy who's on the journey too. When I decided in my 30s to stop attending the church I grew up in, I did so not because I felt any less spiritual or religious, but because I realized that some-how I had internalized this "good" versus "bad" idea so much that it was really hurt-ing me and the people in my life. I spent so many years repressing anything about me I thought might be considered "bad." My mentality was that only perfect people get into heaven, and so I strived for perfection. When I couldn't measure up (and of course I was destined to fail, because perfection is an impossible task), I hid those flaws so that no one would know. I felt like two people: the "good" me I showed to the outside world and the "bad" me I so desperately wanted not to be. I had to unlearn this lesson. Not to sound all Oprah about it, but it's true: I had to learn to love myself—all the parts of me (the good, the bad, and the ugly). Our society doesn't talk about how important this is for men as well as women. With lots of inspiration from Brené Brown's books *Daring Greatly* and *Rising Strong*, I began teaching

myself that all feelings are valid, that we're all human, that it is vital to own our stories, and that real strength isn't in avoiding our flaws, it's in our ability to be honest about our vul-nerability. I even have that tattooed on my forearm as a constant reminder: vulnerability is strength.

I see this same dynamic all the time in the fitness and diet industry, and it's what causes so many of us—myself, Amy, and thousands more—to struggle: we create these catego-ries of "good" and "bad" foods, people, and, activities, and then we align our lives accord-ingly, no matter how difficult or restrictive it may make our lives. There are only two options from this point: we either fail or suc-ceed at following all the rules. But no one can be perfect all the time. You know that, right? We are setting ourselves up for failure when we try to be perfect. That's not what I want for you (or for me). I want to give you a lifestyle that, as one person told me, "just clicks"—where you get to eat food you love and are supported in a journey toward loving foods you used to push around your plate at your childhood dinner table, and where you are empowered and feeling great each step of the way. This isn't dieting, it isn't dogma, it isn't deprivation—it's support, empathy, and community. Loving the journey, not just the destination. Strength in our vulnerability. Own your story!

The following sections are everything you need to know about getting started with keto. Like a compass or a field guide to help you have the best keto experience possible. It's not meant to be the Google Maps voice annoyingly telling you each turn one at a time, even if it's telling you to turn right when there is no right and you're on the verge of throwing your phone out the window. Am I right, or what? It's more like a good old-fashioned map that's there to help you find your own way to your best health. When I start talking about keto dos and don'ts, I'm not giving you a dogma to follow; I'm giving guidelines for you to use in the *context* of the big picture of your life and your goals to help you have an optimal experience.

You are welcome here no matter what, even if you've never thought about your sugar intake a day in your life or if you're a purist and you never touch anything that's a chemical. If your starting point is that you've been living off soda, pizza, and crackers all your life and you feel overwhelmed and intimated by the food list, you are very welcome here. Remember your why—why are you doing this? It's more important to me that you're committed to your personal why than it is that you follow every tip I've laid out in this section.

HOW TO KNOW YOU'RE IN KETOSIS

As you get started with keto, the first thing you'll need to do to track your progress is to find out if you're in ketosis. You'll know you're in ketosis by testing your ketones, which you can do in several ways that I'll explain below. I recommend checking your ketone levels during the first two weeks of my 30-day program. After the program, I recommend you test after eating something

new so you can see how it affects you. I'll talk more about testing for ketosis long-term in Part 4. For now, keep in mind that although I'm going to lay out solid guidelines for your macros and a detailed meal plan for you to follow, keto is very bio-individual. Your hunger levels won't be the same as mine. What affects you might not affect me. Every person is different, and testing will help you learn about your body and how it reacts to certain foods. For me, if I eat a Big Mac from McDonalds without the bun, my ketones drop from 1.0 to .5. Maybe because it's not made of healthy fats, maybe it's something in the sauce. Or it could be the dairy. I know this because I tested in the beginning and I test when I eat something new, like the good self-experimenter I am. That's why you have to test—every person's going to be different.

Knowledge is power and measuring your ketones will help you personalize keto for you. This isn't mandatory, but it's an option for those that want to go up a level when it comes to their health. It takes some self-experimentation, but it does pay dividends, I promise.

Although I recommend that you test, at least in the beginning so you learn about yourself, if you have no interest in testing and just want to follow the meal plan and exercise regimen of this program, you'll still get all the benefits of my program! I know lots of people who don't test at all, whether because they can't afford the testing materials or because they're just trying to lose weight and eat better and don't care about ketone numbers. If you don't test, you can still look for physical signs you're in ketosis that you can use as a guideline. Physical signs may include a slight change in the way your breath smells (due to an increase in a type of ketone called acetone) and an increase in mental clarity. You may also notice decreased appetite and increased energy—or if you have what's called the "keto flu" you may experience nausea, brain fog, muscle cramps, fatigue, and dehydration. Let's all hope that this doesn't happen to you, but if it does, check out my "keto dos and don'ts" in the following pages as well as the section on side effects and how to minimize them starting on page 60.

As one person told me, "I don't feel I need to test because I'm happy to have a plan that gives me delicious, filling food and gives me great results. Plus I know you've done the homework for me!" For some people, it just doesn't make sense to chase ketones if you feel great, you've got a great plan, and your body and mind are transforming. However, if you've decided not to test and you aren't seeing the results you hoped for, I recommend giving testing a try because being in ketosis is crucial for reaping all the benefits of keto.

If you *are* up for some self-testing, I think it's a great way to learn more about your body and what works best for you. There are three ways of testing: your breath, your blood, or your urine. What are you actually testing for? You're testing for beta hydroxybutyrate (BHB) levels in the blood, acetone in the breath, or acetoacetate in your urine—these are three different types of ketone bodies that you'll start producing once you're in ketosis. So how does each test work and what are the pros and cons?

Urine Testing

Urine ketone testing is the cheapest way to test—for around 10 bucks at the drugstore you can get 50 strips. The strips measure the excess concentration of acetoacetate in the urine. There is a color change—the strip turns dark purple—within 15 seconds if ketones are present. If you have ketones in the urine, then your body is producing ketones and you are most likely in ketosis.

PROS

It's the least expensive method for testing ketones. Plus the test is painless: you just pee on a stick.

CONS

Because it only measures acetoacetate in the urine, this method cannot measure long-term ketosis. Why? When you first get started on keto, your body starts producing ketones right away but it's not yet very efficient at using them. So it gets rid of a lot of them in your urine in the beginning. After a while your body gets more used to using the ketones—what we call becoming fat-adapted—so you won't see the strip turn color as much because ketones aren't being thrown out so much as waste in the urine, they're being used by your body! So even if you do not have ketones in your urine, you still might be in ketosis, with ketones showing up in the blood (as beta hydroxybutyrate). The urine test is very useful in the beginning, and less so over time.

Blood Testing

Blood testing is the gold standard and the most accurate way to test the ketone levels in your body. It requires a little finger prick that detects beta hydroxybutyrate. The results are shown with a clear digital display. Anything above .5 mmol (millimoles) means you're in ketosis. Anything below means you're not.

PROS

It's accurate. It doesn't get any better than this if you want clear, accurate results.

CONS

Blood testing requires a blood-ketone meter (which costs roughly $30) and some blood ketone measuring strips (anywhere from $1 to $3 per strip), so it's more expensive than urine testing; especially if you're testing twice a day, the cost of those strips can add up. These supplies can be hard to find in stores, so you may have purchase them online. Perhaps the biggest con, though, is that whole drawing blood part, which is a big deterrent for some. If you do decide to purchase a meter, I use this one found at this URL (where you'll receive a discount, obviously): bestketonetest.com/fit2fat2fit.

Blood testing remains the king of keto testing, so if you can afford it and you can stand the finger prick, I recommend giving this a try. I think it's worth it to make that initial investment to get to know yourself— and then take a break so you don't get too obsessed with the numbers and don't need to keep buying strips.

Some tips if you do go this route: just buy 20 strips and for the first two weeks test to see where your levels are at in the morning and at night, and maybe before and after certain meals, so that you know how certain foods affect your ketone levels.

From there you don't have to test for the rest of your life, unless you want to get another set of strips in three or four months to test again and give yourself feedback and some biomarkers to look into.

Breath Testing

Another popular way is to use a breath-ketone meter (like the one from LEVL). Breath testing is the only way to measure acetone in the breath. It's a pretty accurate method and the tech is pretty cool—it syncs to an app via Bluetooth.

PROS

This method is painless, there's no blood and no needles, plus it's easy to do and you can test anywhere and as many times as you want throughout the day.

CONS

It can produce unreliable results, because although blood ketone and breath ketone levels usually match up well, sometimes they don't. So it's not as accurate as blood testing. You may not want to or be able to blow into the unit for the required 10 to 30 seconds. It's also way more expensive than the other methods: the LEVL device costs about $500 and then you pay about $50 a month to calibrate the meter. The good thing is that the meter is a one-time purchase. The downside is there's an initial investment plus the recalibration every month. But then again, you don't need to prick your finger or draw blood, so that may be worth it for you.

Some people I've worked with have found that they love the urine strips because they're so cheap, accessible, and easy to use; while the results may not be as accurate as blood testing, they've found that it gives them enough information to work from in conjunction with physical symptoms and observable results. Others have shared with me that urine testing just didn't feel certain or reliable enough, while blood testing gave them confidence that they were getting clear results. For some, the blood testing just wasn't at all appealing, and so breath testing was the way to go. The bottom line is that testing can give you lots of information about you, your diet, and your body, so choose which method works best for you. Do urine testing if you want a cheap, painless way of testing whether your body is producing ketones in the beginning of your keto journey; do blood-ketone testing if you are willing and able to spend a little money to get a super accurate reading, don't mind a little pinprick, and want something that will work well over longer periods of time; choose breath testing if you've got some money to invest, and you really want to test long-term and you really don't like needles.

If you choose to do no testing at all, that's okay; you can still see benefits on this program. But if you do want to be as effective as possible, it's important to test at some point.

BEING IN KETOSIS VS. BEING KETO-ADAPTED

Keto is not like other diets where you do it for a few days and then maybe you relax a little bit or fall off the wagon and then you get back to the diet—the longer you stay in ketosis, the more efficient your body gets at burning ketones as an energy source, which means your body is more efficient at using fat for fuel. So if you fall off the diet for a few days and binge for a day or two, you'll get kicked out of ketosis. You're human, it happens. And this can happen with any kind of diet. But with keto, just know that you're probably going to be starting at ground zero when you get back to it.

If you stay consistent for a minimum of 30 days—60 or 90 days is optimal for some people—your body will get *really* efficient, and you'll go from being in ketosis to being what's called *keto-adapted*. Ketosis is a state you achieve by limiting glucose and kicking on your body's backup ketone burning system. When you're keto-adapted your body can switch back and forth between glucose and ketones because it's become so efficient at producing and using ketones. When you've made making and burning ketones very clear for your body, it already knows what to do next time. So if you can stick it out for that first 30 to 90 days, and then you choose to eat carbs for a while, when you go back to keto, your body is going to be able to get back into a ketogenic state faster because it's a familiar state. You've become fat, or keto, adapted.

Think of it this way: If you haven't run for years (or ever), your first day of running is probably going to hurt. Really bad. Trust me, this literally has happened to me. It's going to be hard and it's going to suck. Right? But the more consistent you are at going for a run, the more efficient you become at it, and the fewer calories your body has to burn to do it. With keto it's the same: it can be harder in the beginning because your body is adjusting, but over time your body will become more efficient at it and it will get easier. So be patient with yourself. The longer you do it, the easier and more efficient it will be. Don't expect to run a full marathon if you haven't run in 30 or 40 years—start wherever you are and give yourself the time and space to adjust. On the other hand, if you skip a week or two when you're already a consistent runner, you can go back to running with little difficulty. Getting fat-adapted works the same way; it takes some time, but after time you become more efficient and more practiced and then it gets easier.

KETO DOS & KETO DON'TS

Here are some of my best tips and tricks for living keto as optimally as possible—they're good support for both phases of my program, the keto cleanse in Part 3 and keto for life in Part 4. Think of this as a troubleshooting section; you can refer back to it as you make your way through the 30 days or anytime after. I'm putting it here for you to read now because it gives you a sense of the philosophy of the keto lifestyle, plus it helps you be prepared for what's to come, so that when you start the program you're already armed with lots of information on what to do when things get tough.

Get enough fat

Whenever you're not sure what to eat on keto, eat more healthy fat. Most people struggle with getting in enough fat. Why? Here's the thing: society in the developed Western world is set up to give us protein and carbs. Anywhere you go, getting protein and carbs is really easy. You almost have to go out of your way to add healthy fats into your diet. We've bought the lie that fat = bad for so long that on keto you're a little bit like Matt Damon in *The Martian*—you might feel like you're on another planet entirely. So don't be afraid of adding in healthy fat whenever necessary. Even if your waiter gives you some side-eye, go ahead and ask for extra-virgin olive oil, coconut oil, butter, or avocado when you're eating out. Add it to the meals you make at home. Fat is your friend.

Let me give that one a caveat: fat is your friend as long as you're limiting carbs. Fat itself doesn't put you into ketosis; it's the lack of glucose that does it. So go ahead and add healthy fats, but make sure you're also keeping your carbs low.

While you're keeping your carbs low, though, be careful not to overdo it with alternatives such as keto cookies, keto pancakes, other keto dessert recipes (and trust me, there are plenty; just go have a look at Pinterest), or fat bombs. I don't recommend going overboard with these things because all these keto desserts are very calorically dense, meaning they are very high in calories. It's okay to have them from time to time, but on the daily it's not optimal if you're trying to lose weight, because the problem is that you're still using the same behavior—eating something sweet as a reward or to manage stress. It's best for us to look inside ourselves to figure out why we are eating these foods. What is our intention? Is it a reward? Is it old programming to reach for something sweet when life gets stressful? It's important to understand if these old behaviors are controlling us or if we're controlling them. This is why I offer so much emotional and spiritual support in my program—so that rather than just changing your diet, you can get to the root of your cravings and truly transform.

Drink lots of water

How much should you drink? Divide your body weight by 2 and that's the minimum number of ounces per day you should consume. So if you weigh 200 pounds, you'll want to drink 100 ounces of water a day. If you're working out and you're really active, you definitely need more than that.

It's best to drink it first thing in the morning. Your body wakes up dehydrated after sleep (it's been detoxing all night long while you snore away dreaming of keto cookies), so after you pee, the next thing you should do is drink a lot of water. Have a glass ready to go the night before so that in the morning you don't even have to think. Feel free to add a pinch of sea salt or lemon for optimizing this experience. All you have to do is chug.

If you're saying, "That's too much water, Drew!"—I know, I know, it seems like a lot. Here are some hacks to help you get those ounces in: Buy a bigger cup or get yourself a nice plastic-free water bottle. The environment will thank you. Some people carry around gallon jugs—yes, really!—of water or a large Hydro Flask so that it's easier for them to get more water in that way. You'll find it easier since you don't have to constantly refill the water. Plus measuring in a large container is simpler than doing it cup by cup.

You could also set a timer. Some people need a reminder every now and then to drink. So setting an alarm on your phone every 30 to 60 minutes can be helpful to remind you to drink.

If you find you get bored drinking so much plain water, try flavored water with no sweeteners. Adding in a flavored sparkling water with no sweeteners definitely helps mix things up. Plus there are so many amazing flavors now; there's almost no excuse to not get your water in.

Get your electrolytes

Supplement potassium citrate 1,000 to 3,500 milligrams per day and magnesium glycinate or citrate 300 to 500 milligrams per day while you're on keto. Use these forms specifically because they're the most bio-available, which means they're optimally for-mulated so that the nutrients pass from your gut to your bloodstream—no reason to take a supplement that your body can't even use, right? Okay, I know I said none of these tips are dogma, but this one is not optional. This is MANDATORY. When you start keto, your body will initially get rid of a lot of water—with expelling a lot of water, you also lose a lot of minerals. Think of it this way: What hap-pens if you add water to bread? The bread absorbs the water. What happens if you add oil—fat—to water? It separates. So your body gets rid of a lot of water on this high-fat diet. People tend to lose a lot of water weight on keto, which is awesome. But this also means you're losing minerals, causing an imbalance in your electrolytes, which can result in things like muscle cramps, headaches, and brain fog. If you balance out these electrolytes, you're going to feel so much more optimal during

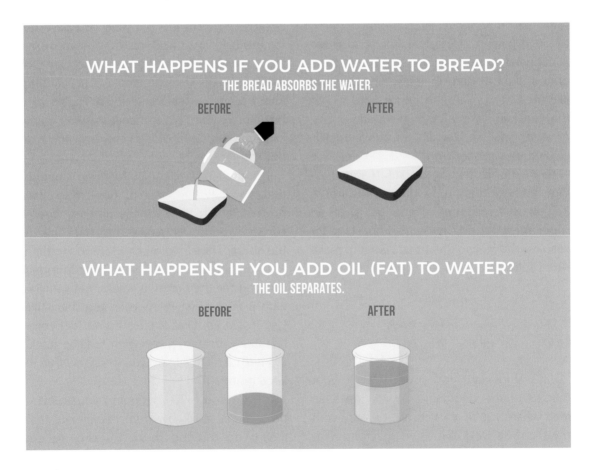

the transition. The transition still might be hard, but these things will help out. They will get rid of 99 percent of problems.

Get enough salt, too

Add sea salt, Celtic salt, or pink Himalayan salt to your food, about 5–8 grams per day. Not white table salt, only sea salt (or kosher sea salt, which is just larger salt crystals than sea salt), Celtic salt, or pink Himalayan, because they are more mineral rich. We definitely demonize salt in the standard Western diet, but on keto you need it. Why? For the same reason as above. Because you're going to be expelling electrolytes like crazy and you'll need to re-up so you don't get dehydrated, lightheaded, or foggy. If you don't like the taste of salt and find it hard to get that much in, take salt tablets instead.

Yes, you can get all the above minerals and electrolytes from food. I've felt fine without supplementing because I was making sure I got them in food form, but in the beginning I recommend you get them in supplement form. They're so important for keeping you feeling great that I want to make sure you're getting all the support you need.

Track your macros the first two weeks of the program

It's important for you to track your macros in the beginning so you have an idea where you're at. This will be easy with my plan, because I've listed macronutrient content for every meal. But in the long run, and anytime you're going off-plan, I encourage you to get curious about reading nutrition labels, where you'll find the amount of total fat, total carbs, and protein per serving (double those numbers if you're having two servings). If you're doing vegan or vegetarian keto, you can subtract fiber content from total carbs to figure out net carbs. You can track this information in a food journal. Or to make things super easy, I recommend using an app like MyFitnessPal that allows you to enter your meal and then calculates macronutrient content for you.

I ask you to track in the beginning because if you're just guessing you have no idea, but if you track you can know you're at 50 percent fat, or if you're eating way too much protein. Tracking is all about learning about foods and learning about you. It can help you realize "Wow, there's way too many carbs in nuts," or "I didn't know avocado had this many carbs."

Once you've done it for long enough that you have an idea of how much fat, protein, and carbohydrates different foods contain, you no longer need to track. Life is too short. There's so much more to life than tracking macros. That's why I recommend tracking for the first two weeks; get familiar with it in the first two weeks and then, like Elsa in *Frozen*, "Let It Go," if you feel comfortable with that. If you want to keep tracking because it's helping you, then feel free to keep going.

The reason I'm cautioning you to let it go is because I know from experience that if you do this too much it's easy to get obsessed. Don't freak out if you're one gram over. Tracking your macros is information, it's not God. You're not going to go to jail, you're not going to ruin everything, the keto gods aren't going to curse you if your macros aren't perfect. It's a journey and a process. Do your best, gather information, and keep on keeping on.

I recommend posting your macros in my Facebook group or wherever your support system is so that you get that sense of community support and feedback. Along with tracking your macros in the beginning, I also think it's a great idea to keep a food journal, especially if this lifestyle is new to you. It's important to know. Knowledge is power! Food journaling, which is basically just keeping track of what and how much you eat, can help you understand food better—"So this is what 1,500 calories looks like!"—and all this information gathering helps you get comfortable reading nutrition labels and be more mindful about what you consume. It's important because you'll start to know and learn what foods are.

But again, don't let it own you or run your life. If after the first two weeks you find you're at a restaurant with friends entering your meal into MyFitnessPal or whatever app and it's taking 15 minutes away from your friends, as Randy Jackson from *American Idol* would say, that's gonna be a no for me, dog. Track in the beginning, but not for the rest of your life. Be with your friends. Be present to your life.

Read nutrition labels for total carbs, not just net carbs[*]

Net carbs are the total number of carbohydrates minus fiber and sugar alcohols, because these types of carbohydrates are thought to have a minimal impact on blood sugar levels. Total carbs are just that: the total number of carbs. You may have heard you can go by net carbs instead of total carbs, and if you've been on keto for a long time and know your body really well, then you know best if calculating by net carbs works for you. But if you're new to keto, it's important to start out with total carbs and use that as your measuring tool for everything. Why? Because certain carbs that count toward total carbs, but would be excluded in calculating net carbs, can still affect your ketone levels. So for now, during this beginning keto cleanse phase, I want you to be on the safe side and stick to total carbs because I want to give you the best possible experience.

Enough Mr. Nice Guy—let me hit you with some DON'TS! Just kidding. These aren't rules I'm going to scream over you while you do 1,000 burpees—I give you these tips to help make your transition into ketosis as supported as possible. On that note, here are some of Drew's DON'TS:

---

* Unless you're doing the veg*n version of my plan. If you're doing veg*n keto, you can go by net carbs so that you have enough to make you feel satiated.

Stay away from unhealthy fats

By unhealthy fats I mean things like margarine, Crisco, vegetable oil, and hydrogenated oils. Anything super processed. This is just a good life lesson: the less processed, the better. Some people use keto as an excuse to eat mayonnaise and deep-fried everything, because these foods are high in fat. Thing is, these fats cause inflammation in the body. Even though the American Heart Association thinks coconut oil is bad but vegetable oil is good, and even though technically on a macro level these unhealthy oils are keto, they're not healthy for your gut and for your inflammation levels. Healthy fats, like coconut oil, for example, have been shown to have antioxidant, anti-stress abilities—and have even been found to be good for heart health.[1] I don't just want you to lose water weight— I want you to optimize your health and your body. So yes, there is a difference—in your gut, your heart, your joints—between margarine and avocado. Pick grass-fed butter, extra-virgin olive oil, and coconut oil over Crisco and make your gut and everything else feel much happier.

Stay away from starchier veggies

Not all vegetables are alike—starchier veggies include things like potatoes, sweet potatoes, beets, winter squash, parsnips, peas, and carrots because they contain higher amounts of carbohydrates than non-starchy vegetables like kale, spinach, broccoli, and cauliflower. If you go heavy with starchier veg, it may kick you out of ketosis, so especially in the beginning you'll want to stick with non-starchy. You'll see that the meal plans I've included emphasize non-starchy veggies, and you can use my menus to guide your food choices.

Be careful with onions—although technically they're a non-starchy veggie, if you caramelize them they'll be higher in carbohydrates. You know how caramelized onions are super sweet and delicious while raw onions are bitterer? On a molecular level, in caramelizing, you've changed the onion from a polysaccharide to a monosaccharide—in other words, from a larger sugar to a simple sugar. And this means it can more easily spike your blood sugar and affect whether or not you're in ketosis. Sometimes certain mushrooms and bell peppers can kick people out of ketosis, too. Remember your keto macros; you're trying to get 75 percent of your daily caloric intake from fat, 20 percent from protein, and 5 percent from carbohydrates. So when it comes to keto, not all veggies are created equal: the lower the carbs, the more you can eat without exceeding your macros. Take a look at how the most common veggies compare in terms of carb content, or high-carb versus low-carb veggies.

LOW-CARB VS. HIGH-CARB VEGGIES

HIGH CARB

1 CUP CHOPPED ONION
= 64 calories, 14.9 grams carbs

1 CUP CUBED SWEET POTATO
= 114 calories, 27 grams carbs

1 CUP CUBED BUTTERNUT SQUASH
= 63 calories, 16 grams carbs

1 CUP DICED RUSSET POTATO
= 120 calories, 28 grams carbs

1 CUP YELLOW CORN
= 125 calories, 27 grams carbs

1 CUP GREEN PEAS
= 118 calories, 21 grams carbs

1 CUP BEETS
= 59 calories, 13 grams carbs

1 CUP CUBED ACORN SQUASH
= 56 calories, 15 grams carbs

1 CUP ARTICHOKE HEARTS
= 94 calories, 22 grams carbs

1 CUP LIMA BEANS
= 217 calories, 39 grams carbs

1 CUP CUBED YAMS
= 177 calories, 42 grams carbs

1 CUP STEWED TOMATOES
= 80 calories, 13 grams carbs

1 CUP SUGAR SNAP PEAS
= 60 calories, 10.5 grams carbs

1 CUP CHOPPED JICAMA
= 49 calories, 11 grams carbs

1 CUP CHOPPED CARROTS
= 53 calories, 12 grams carbs

LOW CARB

1 CUP CHOPPED CAULIFLOWER
= 25 calories, 5.3 grams carbs

1 CUP CHOPPED ASPARAGUS
= 27 calories, 5 grams carbs

1 CUP CHOPPED CELERY
= 16 calories, 3 grams carbs

1 CUP CHOPPED BROCCOLI
= 31 calories, 6 grams carbs

1 CUP CHOPPED KALE
= 33 calories, 6 grams carbs

1 CUP SPINACH
= 7 calories, 1.1 grams carbs

1 CUP CHOPPED ZUCCHINI
= 21 calories, 3.9 grams carbs

1 CUP SLICED YELLOW SQUASH
= 19 calories, 3.8 grams carbs

1 CUP SLICED GREEN BEANS
= 31 calories, 7 grams carbs

1 CUP CHARD
= 7 calories, 1.3 grams carbs

1 CUP ROMAINE LETTUCE
= 8 calories, 1.5 grams carbs

1 CUP SLICED CUCUMBERS
= 16 calories, 3.8 grams carbs

1 CUP SHREDDED CABBAGE
= 17 calories, 4.1 grams carbs

1 CUP SLICED MUSHROOMS
= 16 calories, 2.3 grams carbs

1 CUP BRUSSELS SPROUTS
= 38 calories, 8 grams carbs

No grains, rices, cereals, breads, pastas, chips, cookies, or crackers

Whew! I tend to focus on what you can enjoy on keto—and there's so much!—but sometimes you just have to name the NOs. Can you guess what all the above have in common? Yup, they are carb heavy—or they're carb heavy *and* most likely full of sugar. All carbs turn to glucose in the body; it doesn't matter what the carb is, it gets turned to glucose in the body, and the purpose of keto is to starve the body of glucose as an energy source so that your backup generator kicks in and your body starts burning fat for energy. If you feed your body these carb-heavy foods, eating all the healthy fat in the world isn't going to do a dang thing for you. You have to minimize glucose, and you do that by limiting your carb intake to 30 grams total carbs or less a day.

This is important, so let me repeat it: even though I tell you fat is your friend and to make sure you get enough fat, eating fat alone doesn't make you produce ketones. It's the lack of glucose that forces your body to produce ketones. I get a lot of questions from people saying they haven't eaten the full amount of recommended fat for the day and they're worried they're not in ketosis because they didn't get enough fat—that's not necessarily true. It's the lack of glucose that forces your body to produce ketones. If you're eating high fat and high carbs, your body's going to run off glucose and it's just going to store and hold on to the extra calories from the fat. This is counterproductive for fat loss goals and also for all the health benefits to your heart, hormones, gut, and brain that keto offers. Eat healthy fat, yes, but just as important, starve your body of glucose by limiting your carb intake.

But what about healthy organic cereals like Kashi or diet cereals like Special K? They are carbs—and they're almost always full of sweeteners. Even foods like paleo bread, low-carb bread, or gluten-free noodles are not in my 30-day program because it's so easy to overdo it—or there are things like nuts or sneaky other grains in the noodles—and any of these can kick you out of ketosis. My goal is to get you into ketosis as quickly, easily, and optimally as possible so that you feel great the whole way through. Even "healthy" versions of these foods can hinder that process, so they're out.

Not to mention you can get way more fiber and micronutrients from vegetables than you can from grains. If we're talking about giving your body the most efficient, most optimal energy source so that you can thrive in your life, why bother with a slice of paleo bread when you can have a guacamole burger with bacon-wrapped asparagus stacks? Once you taste the food in my plan, I'm sure you'll agree, but just in case you need more convincing, let's see how grains measure up against veggies.

1 CUP GREEN BEANS

3.7g Fiber

17.9mg Vitamin C

15.8mcg Vitamin K

40.7mg Calcium

27.5g Magnesium

230mg Potassium

1 CUP BRUSSELS SPROUTS

3.3g Fiber

74.8mg Vitamin C

156mcg Vitamin K

37mg Calcium

20.2g Magnesium

342mg Potassium

1 CUP ASPARAGUS

2.8g Fiber

7.5mg Vitamin C

55.7mcg Vitamin K

32.2mg Calcium

18.8g Magnesium

271mg Potassium

1 CUP CAULIFLOWER

2.5g Fiber

46.4mg Vitamin C

16mcg Vitamin K

22mg Calcium

15g Magnesium

303mg Potassium

1 CUP BROCCOLI

2.4g Fiber

81mg Vitamin C

92.5mcg Vitamin K

42.8mg Calcium

19.1mg Magnesium

288mg Potassium

1 SLICE WHITE BREAD

0.8g Fiber

0.1mg Vitamin C

0mcg Vitamin K

0.1mg Calcium

8g Magnesium

61.3mg Potassium

¾ CUP BRAN FLAKES CEREAL

5.3g Fiber

0mg Vitamin C

0mcg Vitamin K

16.8mg Calcium

64.2g Magnesium

185mg Potassium

1 CUP LONG GRAIN WHITE RICE

0.6g Fiber

0mg Vitamin C

0mcg Vitamin K

15.8mg Calcium

19g Magnesium

55.3mg Potassium

½ CUP QUICK OATS

3.8g Fiber

0mg Vitamin C

1.3mcg Vitamin K

18.8mg Calcium

108g Magnesium

143mg Potassium

1 CUP WHITE SPAGHETTI NOODLES

2.5g Fiber

0mg Vitamin C

0mcg Vitamin K

9.8mg Calcium

25.2g Magnesium

61.6mg Potassium

No juices, sodas, smoothies, or protein shakes

Juices—even green juice—are mostly fructose and carbs, and when you take in fruits and vegetables in this form, you're missing out on lots of nutrients, enzymes, antioxidants, and phytonutrients that come from the pulp. People think carbs = bread, but there are other things that are high in carbohydrates, including fruit, beans, and some veggies. Everything has carbs in it; it's just a matter of how much, and whether in the bigger context of your diet it will kick you out of ketosis or spike your blood sugar. That's why I recommend a powdered greens supplement instead of green juice; you're still getting the micronutrients of veggies without the spike in blood sugar.

I don't recommend smoothies and protein shakes for a couple of reasons: (1) You shouldn't need to supplement protein while you're doing keto. It's not a high-protein diet

and you should be able to get everything you need from food. (2) Some types of protein, like whey, are very insulinogenic, meaning they stimulate the production of insulin, so they may kick you out of ketosis because the amino acid composition of dairy in general and whey in particular can give you an insulin response that spikes your blood sugar. This is not always the case with eating dairy, because if your body has to break those foods down, the process is slower and the insulin spike will be less. But with protein powder in a smoothie you have to be careful. (3) I want you to chew your food the majority of the time and to eat real food as much as possible.

However, if you do want to have a protein shake because you're on the go all the time and you need something convenient and quick, add healthy fat to it to slow down the absorption rate of the protein—something keto-friendly, like MCT oil powder (Complete Wellness has an awesome flavored MCT oil powder that tastes amazing in coffee), coconut oil, or full-fat coconut milk. But in general I recommend not to do protein shakes or smoothies.

Say no to sweeteners

If carbs turn to sugar or glucose in your body, what do you think sugar itself turns into? You got it—glucose! It's the same principle: when you eat sweeteners, they will fuel your body with glucose and kick you out of ketosis.

Some studies are showing that whenever anything sweet touches your tongue—no matter what it is, blueberries, cake, or even natural sweeteners like stevia or monk fruit—your brain can see it as sugar and your body can release insulin in response just as if you had sugar. Just the sweetness of something—your body instantly knows it should release insulin! Sugar is the root cause of all kinds of inflammatory issues, too.

One of the biggest questions I get is how to know what sweeteners are keto-approved, and I know that saying no to sweeteners can be one of the biggest challenges of my plan. Have no fear: there is such a thing as keto sweets—keto cookies, keto pancakes, keto fat bombs—and they're delicious. I encourage you not to overdo it with these things, because, remember, I want you to eat real food as much as possible, but they're there for you in the recipe section when you get that craving for something sweet. If you do have a keto treat, here's a list of approved sweeteners and some not-so-keto-friendly sweeteners.

KETO-APPROVED SWEETENERS

Stevia
(If you purchase powdered stevia, it is commonly mixed with other sweeteners or bulking agents that can cause problems like hidden carbs, so read labels)

Allulose

Monk fruit

Sugar alcohols: erythritol, xylitol

Stay away from these sweeteners.
(How crazy long is this list? Sugar is so sneaky!)

THEY ARE NOT KETO-APPROVED

Agave	Crystallized fructose	Honey
Agave Nectar	Dates	Invert sugar
Agave syrup	Date sugar	Lactose
Barley malt	Dextran	Malt
Beet sugar	Dextrose	Maltodextrin
Brown rice syrup	Diatase	Maltose
Brown sugar	Diastatic malt	Maple syrup
Buttered syrup	Evaporated cane juice	Molasses
Cane sugar	Fructose	Raw sugar
Cane juice	Fruit juice	Refiners syrup
Cane juice crystals	Fruit juice concentrate	Saccharin
Carob syrup	Glucose	Sorghum syrup
Coconut sugar	Glucose solids	Sucanat
Confectioners' sugar	Golden sugar	Sucrose
Corn syrup	Golden syrup	Sugar
Corn sugar	Grape sugar	Turbinado sugar
Corn sweetener	Grape juice concentrate	Yellow sugar
Corn syrup solids	High-fructose corn syrup	

You might also see the words "aspartame" and "sucralose" on a label. Technically speaking, some people on a keto diet can consume aspartame and sucralose without it affecting their ketone levels—it varies person-to-person—but people tend to crave more sweets when eating these ingredients and there are some studies showing negative effects on things like gut bacteria, so I don't include them in my program and don't recommend them.

SUPPLEMENTS FOR A KETOGENIC DIET

You don't need many supplements on the keto diet because you're getting almost all your vitamins and minerals from whole foods, and since you're only getting 25 percent of your calories from protein, you shouldn't need to supplement any protein on my program. However, good, well-chosen supplements are key for helping you have the best keto experience possible.

The list below may seem long, especially if you've never taken a supplement before in your life—and I know y'all are out there—but keep in mind that some of the supps I discuss here are optional things you can use for optimizing your experience, some are to help make sure you're getting or exceeding all your nutritional needs so you feel your best, and others are straight up mandatory to support your transition to keto.

With any supplements, be on the lookout for hidden ingredients that could knock you out of ketosis—watch for carb content, protein, and sugars. Remember that you shouldn't need protein powder, but if you do use some, make sure to add fat to help keep the protein from breaking down really quickly in the body and spiking your glucose.

Have I mentioned that sugar is very sneaky? Like that Cookie Crook character always trying to steal Cookie Crisp, it's always trying to creep its way into your food. Added sugar comes in all kinds of names, as we saw above, like honey, agave, coconut sugar, dates, high-fructose corn syrup, and more. And yes, it can even be hidden in your supplements. Keep that list of sweeteners to avoid handy when you're picking up your supps.

Mandatory

SODIUM, POTASSIUM, AND MAGNESIUM

You need to get enough potassium, salt, and magnesium on keto or you'll be losing too many electrolytes and you'll feel like crap. Supplement potassium citrate 1,000–3,500 milligrams per day and magnesium glycinate or citrate 300–500 milligrams per day while you're on keto, and get 5–7 grams of mineral-rich salt, like pink salt, Celtic sea salt, or Hawaiian salt.

POWDERED GREENS

I recommend supplementing with powdered greens because some people don't eat enough vegetables, especially in the beginning when you're just starting to get used to a new way of eating. A good powdered greens supplement is great to cover all your bases and as an insurance policy to make sure your body is getting all the nutrition and micronutrients it needs. Choose a product without added sugar; if it has sweetener make sure it's sweetened with a natural sweetener like stevia, monk fruit, etc. Look at the carb content, too, so you can include it when counting your macros. Complete Wellness Keto Greens is a great product that I highly recommend, but it's also my brand, so I get it . . . I might be a little biased here. I will say, though, that it tastes amazing.

BONE BROTH

Bone broth is very nutrient dense, especially if it comes from grass-fed cows or free-range chickens. It's full of immune system boosting and healing nutrients like collagen that are great for your skin, too! You can have it with meals or between meals as a snack or boost throughout the day. Bone broth helps with electrolytes as well because it's usually pretty salty. If you're vegetarian or vegan, there are some great keto-friendly recipes for veg "bone" broth out there that is just as nutrient dense so you don't have to miss out!

PROBIOTIC SUPPLEMENTS AND FERMENTED FOODS

These are great for gut health and healing. Pretty much every day there's a new study about the importance of gut health and good bacteria in the gut for everything from autoimmune diseases, food sensitivities, and digestive issues to hormones and mental health. Keto is great for gut health, and making sure you get probiotics daily supersizes that healing. Take a probiotic supplement, or if you don't like to take pills, make sure to eat fermented foods like kimchi, sauerkraut, and pickles—just make sure they contain no added sugar. Complete Wellness also has a great probiotic in the form of a "pixie stick" so you don't need to swallow any pills, and kids love it too!

ADDITIONAL RECOMMENDATION FOR VEGETARIANS AND VEGANS

If you're following a plant-based diet, I also recommend supplementing with a methylated B_{12} supplement as well as vitamin D_3.

EXOGENOUS KETONES

Exogenous ketones are ketones in supplement form! *Exogenous* just means external. (The ketones your body makes are called endogenous ketones because they originate from inside your body.) Most exogenous ketones are in the form of beta hydroxybutyrate, which is identical to the ketones in your blood that your body makes, bonded with sodium, potassium, or magnesium or a combination of the three, usually in large amounts—some have 910 milligrams of sodium in one serving—making it bioavailable so your body absorbs it. Usually 30 to 45 minutes after you supplement you'll see a bump in blood ketones if you test.

The most important thing to know about exogenous ketones is that they will put your body in a *simulated* version of ketosis, which is not the same as nutritional ketosis. You won't burn more fat when you take them. There's no fat loss or weight loss advantage to taking exogenous ketones other than you might feel an appetite suppressant effect. You can't take exogenous ketones and then eat a donut and expect to lose all the weight. When you take exogenous ketones, you're basically elevating your ketones, but not necessarily putting yourself in a state of nutritional ketosis. People think I look like Ben Stiller, but that doesn't mean I live in his house and get to cash those big movie paychecks, you know what I mean?

There are some benefits to taking exogenous ketones that have nothing to do with weight loss. Your brain likes ketones as an energy source, so they'll make your brain happy. You'll notice your ability to function is enhanced while taking exogenous ketones. You'll see an improvement in cognitive function and mental clarity. For this reason, I like to take them before a speech or podcast, when I'm fasting, or if I just have a busy day at work, because they allow me to focus more. They're also good for a pre-workout alternate source of energy if you need an extra boost in the gym or as an appetite suppressant.

When you first get started with keto, your body's not making a lot of ketones. It's learning. It doesn't quite yet know how to use them, like a baby flailing, pumping its legs in the motion of crawling but not getting very far. So exogenous ketones can help you transition during the first couple weeks as you shift from glucose to ketones, because you're teaching your body how to use ketones. Think of them kind of like a horse with a carrot—it helps it learn faster.

Exogenous ketones can also help with inflammation, and there are some therapeutic uses for them.[2] I love them and I take them for all these reasons—they're not necessary, but they can be a great boost to your keto journey. Just don't equate them with faster weight loss.

MCT OIL POWDER OR MCT OIL

MCT stands for medium chain triglyceride, which is a very fast-burning fat that gets converted to ketones really quickly. You won't see a bump in ketones as high as you might if you test after taking exogenous ketones because they convert so quickly, but MCT oil and MCT oil powder will give you a good brain boost and work well as an appetite suppressant. You can put them in your coffee, water, food, smoothies, or even cook with them.

Coconut oil is roughly 60 percent MCT oil—MCT oil is basically the concentrated part of coconut oil they're extracting. So you can add coconut oil to your food, coffee, and smoothies too. Your brain likes it. Coconut oil and MCT oil have a laxative effect if you have too much, so if for some reason you get constipated on the diet you can take them to help with those symptoms. The downside is that if you have too much, it might be too much laxative and you might find yourself sprinting to the bathroom, you know? It's happened to me a few times . . . haha. In this case, cut back.

How to know whether to take MCT oil powder or oil? The powder has a little bit of carbs in it, but it tends to be easier on the stomach, so if you're sensitive, build up your tolerance to MCT oil with small servings of the powder.

I GOT 99 PROBLEMS BUT KETO FLU AIN'T ONE: SIDE EFFECTS AND HOW TO MINIMIZE THEM

Have you heard of what they call the "keto flu"? Symptoms include lack of energy, brain fog, muscle cramping, light-headedness, not feeling good, headaches, heart palpitations, and getting tired quicker during workouts. What is happening to your body when you get the keto flu? Well, basically it's the result of not getting enough electrolytes. You know I'm not all about dogma for its own sake, so when I say electrolytes are not optional, I mean it! If you don't get those in you will feel sluggish and you will experience symptoms of the keto flu. You can experience those things anytime during ketosis, so get your electrolytes whether you're 1 week in or 10 weeks in. That will get rid of 99 percent of keto flu symptoms if you do.

To prevent the keto flu and to get rid of it if you feel it coming on, make sure you're drinking enough water. Get your electrolytes, including

real sea salt in your food (not table salt, which is sometimes mixed with sugar, believe it or not!). Celtic salt and Hawaiian salt are great choices because the minerals are still intact so they're nutrient dense: 5–7 grams mineral-rich salt per day. Get your magnesium and potassium, too: 1,000–3,500 milligrams potassium citrate per day and 300–500 milligrams magnesium glycinate or citrate per day while you're on keto. Otherwise you won't feel good.

If you ever experience keto flu symptoms, here's my flu killer—take a salt shot, with a ton of water, or lemon water, as a chaser, and you'll feel optimal. Or try my homemade electrolyte recipe, which you can find in the Recipes section on page 182.

The keto flu is the biggest possible side effect of keto, but you also want to make sure you're paying attention to things like getting all your nutrients and eating whole foods so that you feel as good as possible. If you go extreme in the interest of weight loss or just eating any old junk, you can become malnourished and lack nutrients. Don't go overboard with bacon, cheese, and lower-quality ingredients. You could technically be keto drinking vegetable oil and sugar-free diet cola all day, but are you going to be healthier and feel better? Probably not. That's not safe.

Lower-quality dairy and low-quality fats cause inflammation. Toxins from the animal get absorbed in the fat—if you're eating animals that were grain fed, shoved into a cage, sick and unhealthy, you're getting all those toxins too because you're eating the fatty cuts of meat. You are what you eat—but you're also what the thing you eat *ate*. Make sense? You eat what your food ate, too. So the quality of your animal products matters. Do yourself a favor and do a Google search of butter from a grass-fed cow and butter from a factory-farmed cow and you'll see there's a huge difference. If you're going to make this commitment, might as well go all the way and take good care of your health, your body, your brain, and your future with good-quality whole foods.

DINING OUT AND TRAVEL

As much as possible, I recommend sticking with approved meals for the duration of my CK30 plan. This will give you the best opportunity to get in and stay in a state of ketosis, which is important for getting all the therapeutic and health benefits of keto and for getting your body to be fat-adapted. However, I know it's nearly impossible to eat every meal at home. Many of us have to travel for work, for one thing. But maybe more importantly, food is also a communal experience, and eating out with friends and family, enjoying yourself at birthday parties and picnics, and so many more situations is an important part of feeling connected and loving your life. So if a situation like this comes up during the 30-day cleanse, or if you're ready to think about doing keto long-term (which I'll talk about in Part 4) and don't want to give up takeout forever, I'm here to help you go into these situations with a plan so you can stay keto *and* have fun with your people.

Surprisingly, it's super easy to eat keto on the road, whether you're at a fast-food place or sit-down restaurant. One of the best hacks I know of is to look at the menu before you go out and see if there's a way to customize it to make it keto. Almost everywhere you go you can ask them to customize and it works. Getting protein and carbs in shouldn't be difficult, so your main concern is getting enough fat. Most restaurants cater to "low-fat dieters," not to high-fat dieters. Here are some simple tips when ordering:

➤ Stick with meat as your main meal. So steak, burgers, fish, sausages, bacon, etc. Just make sure it's not breaded or deep fried. Avoid sauces whenever possible, unless it's cream based—alfredo is mostly keto, for example. Definitely avoid barbecue sauce, which will have sugar in it. If you're vegetarian or vegan, sautéed veggies may make up most of your main meal, but be sure to include eggs or tofu (which is increasingly available at fast-food and sit-down restaurants!), filling fats like avocado and coconut, and nut butters.

➤ Go bunless. For obvious reasons, stay away from breads, pastas, chips, rices, and buns. One hack is to get a burger without a bun, add egg, add avocado, add bacon and extra veggies on the side . . . and you don't have to be afraid if they sauté the veggies in oil!

➤ Drink lots of water. Water will help you stay hydrated on the keto diet.

➤ Ask to add extra butter, oil, cheese, avocado, bacon, eggs, guacamole, sour cream, etc. to your order so you can add more fat to your meal. That way if the menu offers only lean meats, or if you order a salad, you are sure to get your fat in.

➤ Nowadays there are plenty of keto convenience foods that you can take with you on the go—like single-serving nut butter packages, keto cookies, crackers, shakes, meal replacements, and fat bombs. I highly recommend getting your calories from meals first and foremost, but I do think there's a time and place for keto snacks every once in a while—being on the go or eating out is definitely one of those times. So take something with you on a work trip so you have something to keep you keto.

What about going out to parties where most likely there will be cake, soda, pizza, and more? First let me say this: I'm a believer in having fun in life, and so it's okay to enjoy yourself in social situations. There's no reason to get stressed out or worked up about going to a party.

The first step, just like with travel and eating out, is to go into it being prepared. If you've decided that you're just going to indulge this time, then please enjoy yourself. If it's your third holiday party in a row and you want to stay on track with eating keto, here are a few tips to help you be prepared for these situations:

➤ If you do go out and you don't want to eat the food, eat before you go. And more importantly, eat some fat so that you go feeling full.

➤ Bring a healthy keto snack/treat for you and others to enjoy. You never know who will like it and will want to do what you're doing. Plus, it'll give you an option to eat something if you do get hungry.

➤ Talk to yourself. Ask yourself if this is the last time you're ever going to be able to have this food. In most instances it's not. There will always be other work parties, holidays, birthday celebrations, visits to this particular restaurant, etc.

➤ Do the best you can with what you have. You can't always control the foods that will be there, so just do the best you can. Reach for the keto-approved meats and veggies if they're available.

➤ Share your goals. If people see you eating just meat, eggs, butter, cheese, and veggies, they might ask what are you doing and it's an opportunity for you to educate and inspire. So go ahead and tell your friends about your lifestyle change. It's always a conversation starter when you tell someone that you're eating a high-fat diet. People are always interested in how that works, and why, and what you get to eat.

IDEAS FOR EATING OUT WHILE KETO

MEXICAN RESTAURANTS

Fajitas without tortillas, no rice, no beans, top with extra guacamole, sour cream, and squeeze of lime.

Beef or chicken salad, no tortilla, no tortilla chips, no rice, no beans, top with extra guacamole, sour cream, and squeeze of lime.

If you're vegetarian, look for egg options, too. If you're vegan, veggies sautéed in olive oil and topped with extra guac is the way to go.

ITALIAN RESTAURANTS

Grilled salmon or chicken topped with butter or olive oil with steamed vegetables on the side. Request side of olive oil or butter to drizzle on vegetables.

Some Italian restaurants may offer "zoodles" (spiralized zucchini). If your Italian restaurant does, you may have zoodles with meatballs or chicken with alfredo sauce or pesto. (Caution to alfredo sauce: ask if their sauce is made gluten free. Some places use flour as a thickening agent; if flour is used it may kick you out of ketosis. If it is not gluten free it is best to avoid. And go with previous options.)

ASIAN RESTAURANTS

Asian restaurants can be tricky since their dishes are mainly rice based and have quite a bit of sugar in their sauces. But there are a few things you can stick with: egg drop soup, chicken lettuce wraps, pepper steak, and sashimi. Tofu if you're vegan. Don't be afraid to request a side of olive oil to drizzle on meat or soy to increase fat.

PUBS

Lettuce wrapped bacon cheese-burger with side salad, no croutons. May have Caesar, ranch, or blue cheese dressing.

Chicken wings with traditional buffalo sauce with carrots and celery dipped in blue cheese or ranch.

Cobb salad, no croutons, with ranch or blue cheese dressing

Pub food is already pretty hard if you're vegan, but look for a big salad or some good sautéed veggies and lots of guac or avocado.

At the end of the day, life is going to happen—what's that saying? "Life is what happens to you while you are busy making other plans"—and you can't go live in a cave to stay away from the temptations of life. So face them with confidence and know that you have control over your fears.

Don't be scared to go out to eat, thinking you're going to "mess up." Remember your why. Remember the community that's rooting for you and helping you stay accountable. And remember that this isn't a religion—it's meant to improve the quality of your life, not make you miserable or make you feel isolated from your family and friends. If you fail to prepare, you've actually prepared to fail. That is so true in so many situations in our life, right? Check the menu out ahead, go in with a plan, bring some of your fave keto snacks, and then don't fear being in uncomfortable situations. You've got this. Plus, you can just throw me under the bus and tell them that Drew, the Keto Guy, said you couldn't eat that non-keto cookie.

FREQUENTLY ASKED QUESTIONS
Here are answers to the top 10 questions I get about keto:

Q. Should I look at net carbs or total carbs?

A. Unless you're vegan or vegetarian, stick with total carbs for the keto 30-day cleanse just to stay on the safe side. Certain carbs not included in net carbs can affect your ketone levels in the beginning and it's too complicated and stressful to learn which ones do and which ones don't—and then it's easy to fall off the program. So avoid that hassle by sticking with total carbs in the beginning.

Q. I'm not hungry by the time my next meal is due. Should I force myself to eat?

A. Do watch out for undereating on keto. High fat plus protein makes you feel satiated for a long period of time, so it can be easy to find you're not hungry and then not get enough calories.

If you're a man and you're eating 1,400 calories or less per day, or if you're a woman and you're eating 1,100 calories or less per day, you shouldn't be doing that for a long period of time. If you're at a calorie deficit for a long time it can slow down your metabolism, affect your hormones, slow down your weight loss, increase your stress and your cortisol levels. You think less calories equals more weight loss, but it doesn't work that way. There are over 30 hormones that affect weight loss, and if they're not communicating with each other properly it can cause weight gain, slow down the weight loss process, and so much more. You need to eat more.

If you find you're not hungry you probably need to change up your macros a little bit—drop your fat slightly, increase your protein, and see if that increases your satiety threshold to where you're craving and hungry more often. Maybe go from 75 percent to 70 percent or even 65 percent fat and increase protein from 20 percent to 25 percent and see if that helps.

But if your calories are good and you still find you're not as hungry as you used to be, that's okay! Remember that keto is such a high-fat diet it is a more satiating way of eating, so finding yourself not hungry by the time you would normally eat your next meal is common. If you're not hungry, and your calories are good, don't worry about eating; simply listen to your body.

Q. I'm feeling very fatigued and weak. Is this normal?

A. Feeling fatigued, weak, and even sluggish can all be symptoms of keto flu. Make sure you're getting enough water, salt, and electrolytes. Take a salt shot with a water chaser and crush those symptoms ASAP!

Q. Are snacks between meals not allowed? What if I get hungry?

A. I discourage snacking between meals on the keto diet. Since keto is a more satiating way of eating, you should not be hungry between your main meals. Eat a good low-carb, moderate-protein, high-fat meal and you will be able to go hours upon hours between meals without snacking. If you are finding yourself hungry between meals, this either means you have eaten too much protein and/or carbs and not enough fat or you just simply didn't eat enough at your last meal. If you're just craving something as a habit, have some bone broth—it will help with your desire to snack plus give you a good immunity boost.

There's a difference between a craving and true hunger. Ask yourself this. Are you hungry enough to eat raw Brussels sprouts and plain chicken? If not, then it's most likely a craving or just wanting to eat out of boredom. If you are, then it's a sign that you're probably hungry and your body is telling you to eat.

Q. I don't like coffee or tea. What can I have instead of the Keto Coffee for breakfast?

A. You can have Keto Hot Chocolate! Check out my recipe for Keto Hot Chocolate in the recipes section. However, if you do not want to drink your meal (though it is quite filling!) you can have a few scrambled eggs (or tofu) topped with keto-approved veggies and avocado instead.

Q. Constipation: what to do?

A. It's fairly common for people starting out on keto to have irregular bowel movements. You're making pretty significant dietary changes, and making changes to what goes into your body will obviously affect what comes out!

If you are experiencing constipation on keto, then you're probably not eating enough fibrous veggies. I don't recommend supplementing with fiber products, because that's not fixing the root of the problem. Try increasing nutrient-dense, fibrous veggies like broccoli, cauliflower, spinach, kale, Brussels sprouts, etc. Then try increasing your consumption of fermented veggies like kimchi, sauerkraut, and/or pickles. If that doesn't work you can also add in a good probiotic supplement as well. Then you can try adding in more MCT oil. Make sure you're taking a magnesium supplement and drinking plenty of water. You could try decreasing the amount of nuts you're eating and adding more water, coffee, or tea. You can also try taking digestive enzymes, which will help you make sure you're absorbing and digesting all the nutrients in your food. And, most of all, add those 30 grams per day of keto-approved veggies!

It's unlikely you'll experience diarrhea on keto, but if you do, the first thing I'd recommend is giving your body time to adjust to eating all the fats. If your stomach is upset one or two days, it doesn't mean you're doing it wrong. But if it does continue, you may want to cut back on coconut oil and MCT. Without dairy you likely won't have this problem, but if you do for a sustained period, it's a good idea to see your doctor.

"Clean eating" may lift the veil on underlying issues you weren't aware of. If you experience symptoms like diarrhea, constipation, or fatigue on keto, it's always a good idea to see your doctor to rule out things like IBS or an autoimmune issue that may be revealing itself as a result of the clean eating you're doing.

Q. If I have a cheat meal, will I have to start all over?

A. The thing about keto is that you're either in ketosis or you are not. Chances are if you have a high-carb meal or more than 5 percent carbs one day, you'll most likely be kicked out of ketosis. So you will have to work your way back into ketosis. Depending on how far you are into your keto journey and if your body is fat-adapted, it might not take long to get back into ketosis. But if you haven't been keto for very long it may take longer.

I'm not saying you can never have a "cheat" meal, but if you are just beginning your journey you need to allow at least 30 days—for some people it may take 60 or 90 days—before your body is fat-adapted and can adjust to more carbs. You can use exogenous ketones to help get your body back into a simulated version of ketosis, but do not rely on these; they are only a tool to help, not the solution. Remember, it's not the same as nutritional ketosis.

VEGETARIAN AND VEGAN OPTIONS

Calling all vegetarians and vegans! Just a little note that if you're feeling left out every time I talk about meat, I want you to know you can still do this! It's a big misconception that keto = all meat all the time. For some people, it does look like that, but it doesn't have to. As I mentioned above, veg*n keto will have slightly altered macros, ranging from 65 to 85 percent fat intake. I've tried this on myself and have asked my most trusted trainers to try it and we were able to achieve ketosis and stay in ketosis. Totally doable. You're going to have to substitute the meat with vegan protein like low-carb tofu, tempeh, TVP, and low-carb protein powder, or eggs and fish if you're okay with those. Flax, hemp, and chia seeds are great sources of protein for those following a veg diet. I'm including a sample meal plan and lots of veg-friendly recipes for you, so please don't feel left out! Everyone is welcome at the keto table!

KETO AND ALCOHOL

A lot of us enjoy a good buzz every once in a while—plus, it's a cultural and social thing: beer during football/baseball/basketball/hockey/soccer games, wine with a fancy dinner or a spa day, toasts to celebrate milestones. But let's be honest with ourselves: no matter how you spin it, alcohol is NOT healthy. It's a toxin. Most of us know that already. We justify it because of football season, holidays, social situations, stress, etc., but we know it's not great for us. You don't get broccoli and kale hangovers.

Even if you can still drink alcohol and stay in ketosis, keep in mind that it can slow down weight loss and fat loss. The liver will start to process alcohol as quickly as possible, which means it's used by the body before all other nutrients, including fat. Having a drink means you're pushing pause on the fat burning process of ketosis while your liver metabolizes the alcohol—meaning there's less fat being burned in the process.

You'll also notice your alcohol tolerance is lower when eating a keto diet, especially if you incorporate fasting. Since someone following a low-carbohydrate diet will have their glycogen stores depleted and will be running on fats instead of glucose, the alcohol will be metabolized by the liver much faster than someone with high glycogen stores to burn through. So overall, I don't recommend alcohol on keto, and I don't include it in my 30-day program. My program is about optimizing your health and your life and biohacking your body—and a good alcohol detox can go a long way in supporting that journey.

I believe it's okay to enjoy life. Just like I believe it's okay to have sugar every now and then, I also believe it's okay to indulge in alcohol a little bit. In the long term, past CK30, if you want to stay keto but indulge every now and then, hard liquors like vodka, tequila, or whiskey and/or a dry wine are your best bets. Even though hard liquors still begin as carb sources, the sugars are changed to ethyl alcohol during distillation and fermentation. They're basically just alcohol and water, so they don't affect sugar and insulin levels like sugary drinks or beers. Drink liquor neat on the rocks and avoid mixers. That means vodka, gin, and whisky of any kind are all fair game. It's the clearer types of alcohol, however, that go easier on the body.

When it comes to alcohol, keep it simple. Limit yourself. Drink plenty of water in between your drinks too. Just like too much of anything—sugar, water, anything—isn't good for us, neither is alcohol. Know your limits. As much as possible, try to go 30 days without drinking alcohol during the CK30 program.

THE BEST OPTIONS FOR ALCOHOL ON KETO

TEQUILA: Not usually made with added sugars or flavorings, so it's a good default zero-carb choice.

WHISKEY, SCOTCH, OR BOURBON: Even though these are dark liquors, they're still zero carb and therefore keto-friendly.

VODKA: Look for straight vodka or flavored vodkas that don't have added syrups or other sugars.

RUM: You'll get a richer flavor the darker it looks, but all forms are zero carb unless they've been flavored.

GIN: Watch out for flavored gins or those made with mixers in cocktails, as they have added carbs.

A lot of chasers and mixers contain added sugars, flavorings, and syrups, but those aren't the only options. Here are some carb- and sugar-free additions:

- ➤ Seltzer water
- ➤ Erythritol or stevia instead of sugar
- ➤ Sugar-free or diet drinks like Zevia (preferably those sweetened with natural sugar-free options like erythritol or stevia)
- ➤ Sugar-free carbonated water

If you're a wine drinker, Dry Farms Wines makes a keto-friendly wine. It contains less than 1 gram of sugar per liter. Go to dryfarmwines.com/fit2fat2fit to get a 1-cent bottle with your order.

OVERCOMING EMOTIONAL CHALLENGES WITH FOOD

The emotional piece of this journey is more crucial to me than your macros because I know how powerful the emotional connection to food is. When I did Fit2Fat2Fit that was one of the biggest lessons I learned. Before I used to think, just stop eating the junk food, put the soda down, eat the healthy food, and just do it, it's not that hard. But now I know this is hard. That emotional connection to food is way more powerful than I ever imagined. It's not as easy as just putting the soda down.

The first two weeks of going from eating macaroni and cheese and Cinnamon Toast Crunch and drinking Mountain Dew to all of a sudden eating spinach, kale, broccoli, chicken, and fish were hell. Literally hell. (Well, almost literally.) And I'd only been eating the mac and cheese way for six months. Imagine if you've been eating this way for six years or six decades, and now you're trying to eat healthy food. Here's the thing: your body is going to go through withdrawal symptoms. Your body wants that food. It *craves* it. It likes the good feeling of a sugar rush or a carb binge. And then when you don't give your body what it wants, it goes through withdrawal symptoms and you get this low feeling. The food doesn't taste as good and you're not as happy and you do feel hungrier. At times like this, remember that you're on the way to feeling much better. There's a physical connection to food that is very powerful and you can't just overcome it by yelling at yourself to put the soda down. You have to

give yourself time and space and good pep talks—it won't last forever, and soon you'll be feeling fabulous!

We have an emotional connection to food, too. We eat certain foods when we feel lonely, bored, and overwhelmed. We eat certain foods to celebrate an accomplishment or because we're just too busy to cook something. Food connects us to family and friends. So if you take your typical comfort foods out of your diet, all kinds of emotions can come up. Anger, frustration, fear, and even defiance. You may even feel at times like you're going through the five stages of grief. I'm not going to sugarcoat it (because sugar isn't very keto) or pretend that our emotional connection to food isn't powerful. It's real and it's hard.

I have so much empathy and respect for this journey because I know it's not easy. I want to help you win all the time, not just by following my meal plans but by supporting your mental, emotional, and spiritual health. Here are some of my tried-and-true hacks for overcoming emotional challenges with food:

1. Not having the food in the house

Make sure the food you don't want to eat is not in the house. Think about it: if you're an alcoholic and you have beer in the fridge, that's going to be really hard to resist. Let me be real with you: if I have a box of Cinnamon Toast Crunch in my pantry, at some point I'm going to give in and eat it. You thought I was not susceptible, huh? I'm human. I know there's going to be a day where I'm tired, stressed out, and hungry and I don't want to make myself healthy food. I just want to say, screw it, I'm going for that cereal. It's so convenient; I can just walk over to my pantry, pour some into a bowl, pour milk over it, and start chowing down on a whole box of Cinnamon Toast Crunch. Or if I come home and there's a box of Samoas Girl Scout cookies sitting on the counter, I'm going to want to eat the whole thing. I know if I just snack on one or two here and there, I'll just want to get rid of it, and the only way I know how to do that is to just finish the whole dang thing.

So don't set yourself up for failure, because at some point you're going to have a moment of weakness. Life is stressful, you can count on that. And if it's as convenient as walking up to your pantry or cabinet and it's just sitting there staring at you, calling your name like "Drew . . . come eat me, please" (insert very seductive-sounding voice here), it's going to be that much harder. But if I have to go out of my way to go to the grocery store to pick up the milk, pick up the cereal, and then come back home, that's so inconvenient. We are a society of convenience. If we make the unhealthy food inconvenient and the healthy food convenient, it makes it so much easier to stick with this lifestyle. Expect that it's going to be hard to make this change, expect that stress and busyness will arise, and set yourself up for success by keeping those foods out of the house. Don't make it harder on yourself than it already is. Be nice to yourself!

2. Meal prep

When it comes to making healthy food more convenient than unhealthier foods, meal prep is king. Just 5 to 10 minutes of meal prep and planning each night is going to help you stay on track. It can be as elaborate as making your meals for the week ahead or as simple as sitting down and deciding what you'll have for breakfast, lunch, and dinner the next day. You can wash and chop vegetables when you buy them so they're right there in the fridge ready to go when it's time to cook. If you say to yourself, "Okay, I'm going to eat keto," and have nothing healthy prepared to bring with you throughout the day and you're just going to "wing it," then when you go to work and people bring in donuts or you have to go out to lunch with your boss and they're going to a pizza place, it's going to be that much harder to stick with it. But if the night before you decide, here's my breakfast, here's lunch, here's my dinner, here's my snacks, and you spend the time to prepare it and bring it with you, you most likely won't waste that food or that money. You're actually going to eat it. So meal prep is probably one of the most important things, because you're setting yourself up for success, you're investing in you.

These are some great ways to help you reach for keto foods when you're tired, stressed, and craving your old comfort foods, but as I've been saying all along, it's not just about food. For me, the keto diet is so much more than just eating certain food and it's so much more than losing weight. It's a whole lifestyle road map. So let's get into some other kinds of emotional support.

3. Meditation

Meditation has changed my life. It's helped me learn to be present in the moment.

If you're totally new to meditation and you're just getting started, you can download a guided meditation app that's free and it guides you through a 5- to 10-minute meditation. Even if you know nothing about it, that's fine, you're starting somewhere.

Look, I get it. I grew up in Western civilization, too. If you've never meditated before and don't know anyone who does, it might seem weird at first—it seems something that monks do, and definitely not something a fitness keto guy should be telling you to do. But it's not just for levitating gurus in the caves of India anymore—80 percent of CEOs have some kind of meditation practice. People like Tim Ferris, Joe Rogan, and Arnold Schwarzenegger do it. Why? Because it makes you perform better during the day. You're investing in your mental health. If the Terminator can meditate, so can you.

Why be more present? So when you're out and about doing stressful things you can still be present in the moment and not be stuck in the past or worrying about the future. You can see the present moment for what it is. You're going to enjoy the time you're spending with your kids rather than being on your phone. Whether you're with your family, at work, with your spouse, etc.,

instead of worrying about what's going to happen, you'll be more present and at ease.

There are so many applications for a meditation practice in our society. It's becoming more mainstream—I'm willing to bet the people you look up to probably meditate. It doesn't have to be this weird thing where there are chants and incense and statues—although there can be if that's what you like and you practice best that way. You don't have to be a hippie to meditate. And meditation doesn't replace your form of prayer—it's about living in the moment. Don't look at this as a replacement for religion but as a supplement.

The benefits of being mindful and being present in the moment are many—psychological, emotional, and physical. Meditation has been shown to dramatically reduce stress—both increasing general feelings of well-being and also acting as a "buffer" to all the inflammation and neurological damage stress can have on our bodies.[3] It doesn't matter who you are; in this world that we live in, you're going to be stressed out. We all have stress, and meditation is a great tool proven to be effective at reducing stress levels. Even if you are eating healthy food and you're exercising every day, if you're not managing your stress you're not going to see the results that you want to see.

It also helps you be more mindful of what you're eating. So many of us are on our phones while we eat, or we're yelling at our kids, watching TV, answering emails, and more, and we're never truly present with our food. Then food is just fuel for our bodies, nothing more. But if we can be present and be grateful and really taste the flavors and chew it, we'll have such a better connection to it. Mindfulness with our food has also been shown to lead to better digestive health, which helps with overall health as well.

Lastly, it can actually lead to better workouts. Yep, you heard that right. Being good at meditation can help you see better results in the gym. How that happens is through the improvement in the mind–muscle connection. Now that you've learned to be present in the moment and you've become better at breathing, you can feel those muscles contracting that you want to contract during your exercises, which leads to more efficient and safer workouts. Who would've thought that meditation can improve your results in the gym?

Meditation has also been shown to help insomnia, offset age-related cognitive decline, and it can even heal PTSD. Combine all that brain healing potential with the brain happy keto program and we're talking about some major goodness for your body and mind.[4]

Implementing meditation 5 to 10 minutes a day or more is going to pay dividends in so many ways on your physical health. There is a parallel between emotional health, physical health, and spiritual health that for me is at the heart of the keto lifestyle. I don't believe you can reach optimal health without mindfulness, and it can make the emotional ups and downs of any diet, and all the rest of your life, feel much more manageable and even joyful.

4. Practicing gratitude

It's so easy to feel we don't have enough—not enough time, money, shoes, love, friendship, attention. It's like we're all just trying to get through a really stressful week, but every week is like that. We can get caught on a hamster wheel running from one thing to the next and never looking at what we've already got. Diets too often feel this way: like a laundry list of what you can't eat, and you're just pushing yourself through the misery to the end where some magically perfect version of you awaits.

You can get off the hamster wheel to nowhere. You can enjoy your life—and your food—now. Meditation helps with that, but so does practicing gratitude. You can love the journey as much as the destination. You can keep a journal and every day write down three things you're grateful for or that you're proud of. Maybe it's saying no to pizza, cake, or soda. Or even better, maybe it's saying yes to taking a walk. Maybe you're grateful for the food you are eating, not labeling it good or bad, but enjoying the color, the taste, and the texture. Maybe you're grateful for the air in your lungs, a hug from your daughter, or the farmers who grew your spinach. That emotional connection to food—the reason it becomes unhealthy is because we look at food as almost like a religion, like this food is good, this one is sinful, bad, evil, but it's so good I want it. Get rid of that perception. You can change your perception, and if you change your perception you can change your story. If you change your story you can change your happiness. I believe that 100 percent. The more we practice gratitude, the easier it is to look at things throughout the day and have a positive outlook.

5. Positive affirmations

Saying positive words out loud to yourself has power. There are actually studies where they compare saying nice things to rice and plants and saying bad things to rice and plants—the rice and plants that were told nice things grew better and stronger. Now if our words affect how other living things grow, imagine how they affect ourselves at the cellular level. If we're saying positive things about ourselves to ourselves, even if we don't believe it at first, it is really powerful.

Maybe you already have a practice that includes affirmations to develop positive beliefs. Or maybe you're thinking of that *SNL* character Stuart Smalley staring at himself in the mirror, saying, "I'm good enough, I'm smart enough, and doggone it, people like me," and the whole thing is a pretty hilarious punch line—but it doesn't have to be cheesy. Try it for 30 days during the program and see how it feels—maybe at first it's just noticing the negative things you're saying and then eventually replacing phrases like "I hate my thighs" or "I'm so stupid/lazy/fat/whatever" with a positive phrase, such as:

➤ "I'm proud of who I am."

➤ "I love my body."

➤ "I am blessed and healthy and strong."

If these are too hard to say, you could use something like "I'm proud of myself for making this effort," which might feel truer in the moment.

Maybe you say the same thing over and over, or maybe it's five different things every day. What matters most is that you say it out loud or you look at yourself in the mirror while saying it. Or try this idea from my good friend Christine Hassler, who's a life coach. Find a photo of you from when you were a little kid. Take a good long look at that kid. The way you talk to yourself now, would you talk to yourself as a kid that way? Would you say those mean things to that kid? Say your habitual negative things out loud to that child—how does that feel? What positive things would you say to your 10-year-old self?

I love this practice because it shows how mean we can be to ourselves when we would never be that mean to a child or a friend. Why are we so hard on ourselves as adults now? Because society tells us to be that way. We're almost like animals in a circus; we think, if I shock you or whip you, then you'll learn to perform better, but that makes no sense. Not for circus animals and certainly not for us. We've been trained to beat ourselves up thinking that's the way to better ourselves. I think a lot of people have internalized this without even knowing it. I know I did. So our words have power, and if we can have a consistent practice of positive affirmations we can heal a lot of wounds.

These practices—meditation, practicing gratitude, and positive affirmations—helped me transition from growing up hating myself to learning to love myself. It didn't happen overnight, but consistent practice helped me overcome a lot of insecurity, self-doubt, and pain. Even though I was in great physical shape, emotionally and spiritually I was in a bad place, and those things helped me find more balance in life with my mental, emotional, and spiritual health. I'm not just saying these things from a generic place because studies show them to be true, I'm sharing them with you as my own personal testimonial. These little things—five minutes of meditation a day, one positive affirmation a day, practicing gratitude for the food on your plate—they really add up.

Think of your keto experience as a journey, not a destination. Don't let this new lifestyle stress you out, because if it stresses you out it can do more harm than good. Stress increases cortisol levels, which can affect your sleep, your hormones, and more. So these practices are meant to help you not stress out so much. And remember to keep it in context—yes, blueberries have sugar in them, but if you really want blueberries, then go ahead and have a few. You'll be okay. It's not that blueberries are "bad"—it's just that you want to think about quantity.

Don't feel like you have to force any of the meals. If you're not hitting your numbers, you don't need to down a bunch of coconut oil just to hit the numbers. If you're full and you're good and you're not exactly at 75 percent fat or 20 percent protein, it's okay. As long as you keep your carbs under 30 grams, the protein and fats should be okay. You're going to be all right, you're still on track. This is a learning process. The way I do keto now is different from the way I did keto two years ago—I'm constantly learning, growing, and tweaking and that's how it's meant to be. What's most important is that you keep moving forward!

As you turn to the next section and get started on my 30-day program, I want to reinforce that you don't need to chase the numbers. Don't let the practice of having to track everything stress you out to where you freak out if you're one gram over on carbohydrates. Don't let the numbers define you. It doesn't have to be perfect all the time, it's about progress. And remember: You can do this; you can do hard things.

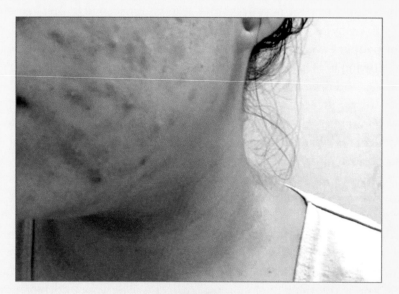

BEFORE

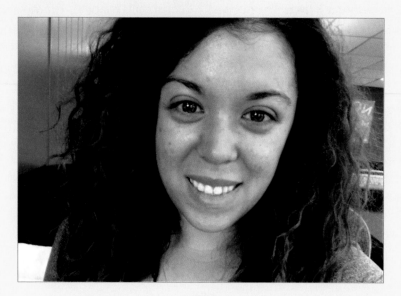

AFTER

STEPHANIE ROEBUCK

I HAVE USED EVERY EXCUSE IN THE BOOK FOR WHY PROGRAMS HAVEN'T WORKED for me or why I can't eat better to lose weight and live a healthier lifestyle. I have been on so many "diets" and "programs" that have failed me completely, so discovering Drew Manning's Keto Jumpstart program has been the best lifestyle change I have ever made! I began my journey after researching keto for several months, for I am the kind of person that requires all the information before taking the leap on anything. Within days of starting keto I started feeling better, eating better, and my skin started clearing up! I have suffered with acne since having my children and have tried countless products, doctors, and medications that never worked for me. I couldn't believe the changes that I was beginning to feel within such a short time frame. I had the energy to go to the gym, play with my kids more, confidence to walk out in public without makeup and even get back into the kitchen cooking (keto cooking now, which is my passion). I am finally back into pre-pregnancy clothing and look even better now than I did back then. I can't believe it! Eating this way is a routine and my chosen way of life. It's delicious and never feels restrictive, which I believe is important in any dietary change. I am forever keto and forever grateful.

— STEPHANIE ROEBUCK

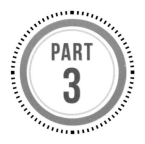

PART 3

PHASE ONE: CK30

I was talking recently with my friend Lauren, who was having a bit of a diet crisis. Her dietician put her on a four-week detox to see if that would clear up some food allergies and stomach issues she'd been having—a no-sugar, no-sweeteners, limited-fruit, limited-carbs, high-vegetable detox. At her four-week appointment, where they were supposed to start talking about reintroducing foods, Lauren was feeling good but not great, so her dietician asked her to do another four weeks. It was overwhelming, she said, but she was committed.

By the end of week eight, Lauren was ready to be *done.* She'd missed having cake on her birthday, she said, and she'd missed candy at Easter. She was missing going out to eat with friends and family.

Then, the day before her eight-week appointment, Lauren's dietician canceled because she'd come down with a cold. "I pulled myself together and made it another five days on this detox and today, the day before my rescheduled appointment, my dietician had to cancel again because of a family emergency! I'm a mess," she told me. "My mental health is really starting to suffer. How can I go another week?"

"Why don't you start reintroducing foods on your own?" I asked her.

"Because I'm afraid I'll do it wrong," she replied. "I guess I don't feel I have the authority."

This happens all too often with health and our diets, doesn't it? We give away our power. We become perfectionists who see ourselves as sick or dependent or defective and we think (hope) someone else will "fix" us, so we stop listening to our own inner authority and give it over to a dietician, trainer, or other health care provider, forgetting that those people are human beings, too, and that the best expert on us is *us*.

What's really going to happen if my friend reintroduces tomatoes on her own? If her stomach issues come back, then it's taught her she needs to stay off them for now. If she feels fine, she's good to go. All that this will give her is *information*; she's not going to die, she's not going to be punished, she's just going to learn more about herself. And that's a good thing!

This is why I'm such a big proponent of self-experimentation—because of Lauren's story and so many others, including my own. We've been taught to worship at the altar of diet and fitness culture, but who ever asks us to look within? No one else lives in our bodies, no one knows how we feel or what works for us better than we do. No expert can tell us what's right or wrong for us. It's true!

Maybe that feels like a lot of responsibility, to be our own health experts, but for me it also feels like freedom—the freedom to be human, to make mistakes and try new things, to be curious about my body and my health without getting attached to ideas of absolute "right" and "wrong."

Why is my Complete Keto program different from every other 30-day keto program? Because I'm not going to tell you that you have to do things my way or hit the highway; I'm here to give you a ton of great meals, workouts, and guidance and then empower you to be your own self-experimenter so that you can find what's optimal for *you*.

All the lessons I learned from my Fit2Fat2Fit journey—the importance of self-experimentation, the need for empathy, honesty, and forgiving yourself when it comes to making big changes, and the awesome power of community—is in this program. So is my experience on *Dr. Oz*, my own personal keto testimonial, all I've learned over the years interviewing all kinds of experts on this diet and lifestyle, and everything I've learned through my personal journey about the importance of tying in the mental and spiritual along with the physical. All of this is missing in the fitness/keto industry—that the power's in your hands, and that you're more than just a number on a scale.

I've put all this wisdom and experience together so that I can set you up for success in every way possible—physical, mental, and spiritual. I know it's not easy to make diet and lifestyle changes, but I also know you can do it. You can learn to trust your own voice. You can find your community. And you can make changes. Your health is worth it—to me, to your family, to your friends, and to *you* so you can get the most out of life.

The program you're about to embark on isn't full of a bunch of B.S. that looks good on paper but makes zero sense for your real life. You can do the CK30 program, including the tough first week, in the context of your normal life, working, parenting, etc.—you don't need to do a home retreat or anything like that. You don't need a bunch of special exercise equipment or cooking utensils. I've walked this walk, and I've walked it with lots of people, everyone from elite athletes to people who've never stepped foot in a gym, and from CEOs to stay-at-home dads. People like Mike, who wrote me to say that "nothing ever truly fit the way your Keto program did, Drew. The food was delicious, and I was no longer ashamed of being someone who needed the help of a diet. I felt empowered to cook more, take charge of my health, and enjoy my life." Empowered—yes, please! Taking charge of your life—yes! Saying good-bye to shame and getting help when you need it—YES!

People like Jeff, too, who shared with me that like most people he started doing keto to lose weight, but looking back on his keto experience he found that that was the least important part. And the most important parts? "Learning to forgive myself for past times of trying and failing, learning that it's not selfish to take care of myself because I deserve it, and the energy I now have to run around with my young daughters." Forgiveness, self-care, and self-confidence, plus a boost of energy to enjoy life? That's what I'm talking about. All this and so much more is the beauty of my program—I'm so excited for you to get started!

As you scan through the program in the following pages, you'll notice that my plan avoids dairy and nuts. Why? Because one of the biggest issues I see is people thinking keto means they can eat unlimited amounts of butter, cheese, and salted cashews—and don't get me wrong, salted cashews are delicious, and cheese and heavy cream at every single meal tastes really good. But overdoing dairy and nuts can stall results. I've seen it time and time again. It stalls weight loss and keeps people from enjoying the full benefits of keto. Dairy is delicious, but it can cause inflammation in the body, especially if you're buying lower-quality dairy products. It can inflame the lining of the gut and cause some gut health damage. Plus, a lot of people—about 65 percent of the population—are lactose intolerant and they don't even know it![1]

Sure, nuts are good for you, but they are very high in omega-6 fatty acids, which studies have shown to be inflammatory. And when the nuts are roasted in vegetable or canola oils, which are also highly inflammatory and not healthy for you, eating them can keep you from experiencing all the benefits of keto as well. Not to mention both dairy and roasted (and salted) nuts are so easy to overeat. You've seen the way a cheese plate gets demolished at a party, right? Not to mention that everything these days seems to come in a three or four cheese option only. Four cheese pizza! Five cheese grilled sandwich! Remember the good ol' days of just mozzarella cheese on a pizza? And have you ever tried eating just a few roasted almonds? Impossible. So these things are easy to overdo and can cause more inflammation in the body, and then you won't feel as great as I know you can.

If you're panicking right now about the no dairy thing, take a deep breath: after the 30 days you can implement dairy and nuts back into your keto lifestyle, don't worry! It's not like you can't ever have those foods again. (And for you vegans and vegetarians out there panicking about the no nuts thing—I know how y'all love your almond milk!—turn to the section that starts on page 126 to see specific info for you.) Think of CK30 as a cleanse or a detox. Cutting out dairy and nuts and following my plan for 30 days is going to give you the most bang for your buck—it's going to give you the best keto experience in 30 days you can possibly get because we're taking out the two most problematic foods that people tend to overeat on the keto diet. Just for 30 days. It's not forever. I'll teach you how to reintroduce those things in a more balanced way after the 30 days so that you can learn how they affect you—just another step on the journey to becoming an expert on *you*.

FITNESS FOR WHEN YOU ARE IN KETOSIS

There is also a workout component to CK30, but before I get into how that works, I'm going to say something else that will probably seem unique among keto programs: I want to stress how unimportant exercise really is when it comes to seeing results. I hear you saying, "What the heck are you talking about, Drew? The only way to get a six-pack is to do crunches all day."

And to a certain extent, of course exercise is beneficial. But what I want you to know is that when it comes to weight loss and fat loss, exercise is not the biggest piece of the puzzle.

Much more important than exercise is staying consistent with your nutrition, getting good sleep, and managing your stress. Doing these things will give you more results than if you exercised hardcore two to three times a day, beating yourself up, straining and depleting your hormones, and messing up your metabolism. I've talked with lots of trusted dieticians who've told me of clients who actually lose weight when they exercise *less*—but nourish themselves *more* with hormone-balancing foods and focus not on pushing themselves through hardcore workouts but on managing their stress. Sounds too good to be true, doesn't it? But I've seen it work myself.

So yes, there is a workout component to my program, but first things first: if it seems too intimidating to do the workout part of this 30-day program, feel free to just go for a walk every day instead. Get up and move every single day. It doesn't have to be a structured 3-sets-of-10-for-16-minutes type of workout, and it doesn't have to be 60 minutes of cardio.

Yeah, you're not going to get ripped and shredded with big, bulky muscles walking for 30 days, but I promise you there will be so many other benefits for your body, mind, and soul in terms of your overall health and your stress levels. Getting outside in nature (even if you're in the city and "nature" is just the sky and a sad little sidewalk tree!) is good therapy; you'll get your body moving, you'll get some good vitamin D and some air, and all of this is more beneficial for your hormones than if you sacrifice your sleep waking up early every morning to hardcore exercise.

Now, if you do want to get into an exercise program to maximize the results of the 30-day program, I've got the program for you! It's a progress-based exercise program, which is unique because it means that you compare your results week to week so that you can track your physical fitness progress and see the progress you're making by a measure other than the scale. The workouts are primarily body-weight exercises, and I designed them that way so you can do them at the gym or at home. Plus, these types of workouts will give you the most bang for your buck when it comes to maintaining lean body mass and burning fat.

I've specifically designed five days of workouts to be repeated Monday through Friday over the course of the four weeks. Saturdays and Sundays are "off" or "rest" days—go for a walk, do something fun and active with your family, maybe take a restorative yoga class. You'll perform all of the workouts during Week One, record your time/score, and then you'll have your baseline. Then you'll compare Week Two results to Week One with the goal of beating your score/time each day.

For example, Monday's workout is an AMRAP, which stands for "as many reps as possible." You'll perform the workout, tally up your total number of reps, and

then come next Monday, you'll try and beat that score—and so on and so forth for the remainder of the four weeks. I use this structure over the four weeks to show you how much stronger and faster you can become if you stay consistent. Each week I'll remind you to go back and compare those results: compare Week Two to Week One, Week Three to Week Two, and Week Four to Week Three—but also compare Week Four to Week One to see how far you've come from start to finish!

My workout program is designed to help you see your own progress so that you can celebrate how far you've come rather than beat yourself up for how far you still want to go. So maybe some weeks you don't lose any weight but you improve your time on a certain workout by 30 seconds or you improve your reps on a workout by 20 reps. Great! This means you're getting faster, you're getting stronger, and you're getting more fit. Heck yeah!

So keep this in mind over the 30 days—progress over perfection. Make it your mantra. Sometimes—often!—the progress you're making doesn't correlate to results on the scale. You might be building lean muscle mass while you're burning fat, which based on the scale would mean you're maintaining or even gaining weight. Scale weight is not God; it's not even Moses. It's just a number. So don't worry about scale weight—think more about what I call "non-scale victories," things like how you feel, how you're sleeping, if you're trying new things, if your clothes are fitting differently. The scale will take care of itself over time. Focus on doing the healthy habits during this program. If you're doing the workouts, that's a healthy habit. If you walk every day, that's a healthy habit. If you stay on track with the meal plans, that's a healthy habit. If you're doing the affirmations and meditations, that's a healthy habit. Let the results take care of themselves; just focus on the process.

MEDITATING

We've all heard of the amazing things meditation can do for us, and you may already have a regular meditation practice (go you!), but it's also possible that you don't meditate at all, or at least not on a regular basis. I think we often struggle to meditate because we feel we need to reach a level of bliss while we do it, and if we don't achieve that (immediately!) we feel like we've failed. But this instant bliss thing is a misconception. Meditation isn't about achieving bliss while you meditate, it's about how you act in your life *outside* of meditation; it's about achieving bliss in your life when you're stuck in traffic, or you're at the grocery store and the person in front of you is annoying you, or your kids are driving you mad. It's about what you do in those moments when the habit of meditation starts to pay off in the rest of your life. Meditation isn't (just) something for monks who've abandoned society and trained their whole lives; it's us in our regular everyday lives—at home, at work, with our in-laws, wherever—being present and not reacting (or overreacting) to everything that comes up.

Another common misconception about meditation is that it means just sitting there not thinking about anything. Let me let you in on a little secret: it's not about not thinking. That's not the goal. The goal is to focus on being in the moment, being present. Paying attention to sounds, smells, sensations, feelings in the body, and breath. Being really attentive to where you are right now—rather than letting your racing thoughts about making dinner, writing a mental to-do list, thinking about all the laundry, be the boss of you.

During my CK30 plan, I'm asking you to meditate every day for 5 to 10 minutes. Throughout the program you'll see a daily space to put a check mark when you meditate and a space to write down your time spent meditating so you can follow your own progress. If you've already got a meditation practice, then please keep doing what you're doing. If you're new to meditation, I recommend that you download a guided meditation app to help you. I really like and personally use Headspace; I also recommend Calm and Brain.fm. I like to rotate between those three. Insight Timer is another good one—they have lots of different kinds of meditation you can try. Just a word of caution: they're all free at first and then eventually they're going to upsell you to more advanced modules. So go ahead and try them all and see what you like best.

Depending on which one you download, these apps will guide you in various ways, but for the most part they're all going to teach you how to become the observer of your thoughts instead of you chasing your thoughts. Headspace does a good job of painting a picture of your thoughts as clouds in the sky, and you, the observer, do not chase the clouds. You see them come and go, but that's the key—they come and go. Just like the thoughts in your head. Then you start to think, "Okay, I'm thinking about X, but let that thought be a cloud that passes by while I focus on the blue sky." The clouds are just going to be here, they're always going to be here. So it's not about not thinking, it's about not getting all attached and reacting to those thoughts; you just see them come and go. And now I sound like Bob Ross with his happy little clouds! Oh, well, I gotta embrace it—meditation is so good for you that it's worth it to sound a little woo-woo for a minute! I promise you'll start noticing results pretty quickly if you stick with it.

You don't need any fancy props to meditate, but if buying a meditation cushion or burning some incense inspires you to do it, then please do. Most important, and most simply, be in a comfortable position—on the floor, on a chair, lying down (but careful you don't go to sleep!), wherever you can feel most relaxed. Lean up against something if sitting up for 5 to 10 minutes is uncomfortable. It doesn't have to be inside, either. Try different places—if you do your meditations indoors for a while, why not change it up and get outside for some sunlight and air? You can do a walking meditation, where you spend time walking quietly in nature, listening to the sounds around you, taking deep breaths,

and being attentive to the present moment. Or, if it's very cold where you are and heading outside doesn't seem like a good idea, maybe try your meditation near a window, next to some good oxygen-producing, air-cleaning plants. You could also just sit outside in a comfy chair, put your earbuds in, and use your app that way. Meditation can be done anytime, anywhere, so don't be afraid to be creative and find a spot that makes you most at ease!

If you're saying to yourself, "I don't have any quiet time or downtime to do this, Drew! How can I meditate when my house isn't clean, the kids won't leave me alone for that long, I have to work all day," or whatever else comes up for you. I hear you. We are all so busy all the time. But let me say this: if we wait for the conditions to be "perfect" to meditate, then we'll never do it. And that's not the point of meditation anyway. The point isn't to achieve perfection, to stop thinking, or to have a super chill life. It's to practice being present amid all the chaos that life has to offer! You're embarking on this Complete Keto journey because you're worth it—nourishing yourself with delicious keto foods is great, but also nourish your mental health, too!

POSITIVE AFFIRMATIONS

I'm also asking you to do a daily positive affirmation during my 30-day program. If you're a beginner to saying positive affirmations and you have no idea where to start, I've included some ideas of what I do to get you up and running for the first week of the program. The first two days of the first week go into detail about how you might come up with an affirmation and some samples for you to try on. The last five days of Week One offer specific affirmations for you to say. You'll want to make your affirmations words and phrases that apply to you in your life. Customize it to your needs. What do you need to hear? What are your negative thoughts and what sentence or phrase can counteract that?

Say these affirmations out loud to yourself. Start with the ones that I offer to get a feel for how it all works, and then for the rest of the program I encourage you to come up with your own that are tailored to you.

It may feel silly at first, if you're new to this, but trust me, I know from my personal experience that this practice works wonders. You may not even realize the negative tapes that are constantly playing in your head (do people listen to tapes anymore?). A few minutes of feeling a little silly by saying positive affirmations out loud has a powerful impact on changing those tapes, giving your mental and physical health a big boost.

FASTING

My program is also unique in that I implement an optional 24-hour fast for Days 1 and 30. Remember that if you starve your body of food, its natural backup system will kick in and you'll be in ketosis. Sweet! So the quickest way to get into ketosis is to stop eating. If you want to get into ketosis, no matter who you are, your age, your weight, your typical diet, or your exercise habits, if you stop eating, you'll go into ketosis. You won't die, you'll just go into ketosis. Promise. Fasting helps get you into a state of ketosis safely and quickly, and this is a great way to jump-start your 30 days—and then jump-start the rest of your life at the end of the program!

The way ketosis works is that in the first two or three days your body is going to start producing ketones, and this transition can be tough for some people. Your body is transitioning, and that can be a little like me trying to get my seven- and nine-year-old daughters to go to bed on time. It will happen eventually but may take some time and extra effort, you know? Symptoms of the keto flu can set in if you're not watching your electrolytes and water. But after about a week or two your body starts becoming more efficient at using those ketones. The whole program is 30 days, because at the end of 30 days, you should start being really efficient and adapted to using ketones as a fuel source. Remember that the goal is not just to get into a state of ketosis, but to become fat-adapted. Incorporating a day of fasting at the beginning and the end helps you achieve that goal. You can expect really good benefits from the 30 days because fasting helps your body get into ketosis really quickly.

Beyond getting into ketosis fast, there are lots of benefits to fasting. Physical benefits include increased resistance to age-related diseases, increased cellular stress resistance and reduced cell damage, and enhanced brain function.[2] It can lower risk for cancer and diabetes and prevent metabolic diseases.[3] It helps lower insulin levels.[4] It's also great for your heart—it improves cardiovascular function and even decreases some risk factors for coronary artery disease and stroke. One study even showed that the results of fasting are similar to those of regular physical exercise![5] It can help improve digestion as well. Convinced yet?

If you're not persuaded by all the many physical benefits of fasting, there's also a mental component to fasting—knowing that your body can go 24 hours without food and you can still function as a human being is very empowering, I've found. You don't need to curl up in the fetal position sucking your thumb, waiting for the 24 hours to be over with. You can be a mom, be a dad, take the kids to soccer, pick them up from school, go to work, jump on phone calls—all those things you have to do in a day. You can still function throughout the day even though there's no food in your body. Knowing that you have that capacity for mental discipline, knowing that you're in control, and your body doesn't control you, it can be profoundly inspiring. You're kind of showing your body who's boss a little bit.

Just for a short period of time. And it gives you a lift that helps you go into the next 29 days with confidence, knowing you have the mental strength to decide for yourself that your cravings don't define you.

For me there's a spiritual aspect to fasting, too. It's been around for centuries and practiced by almost every major religion that exists. There's a component of getting more in tune with your body and more in touch with your spirit or soul. Eating every single day, multiple times a day, for thirty, forty, sixty, seventy years or more, you're just sort of mindlessly putting food in your mouth. You don't often think about what nourishment means, or how your body works, and mindless eating is so often a way of distracting us—avoiding or indulging our feelings, soothing ourselves with sweets, gorging ourselves when we feel stressed, and so much more. When you fast, you get more in tune with your spirit and soul because you're more in tune with your thoughts and feelings, since you can't quickly divert them with cake or pasta. Fasting is a break from just mindlessly eating food. It helps you get in touch with your cravings, your needs and wants, and it empowers you to overcome them or look past them and get comfortable with *you*!

These physical, mental, and spiritual aspects to fasting are the why behind it—it's about more than just weight loss. It's about really making this 30 days a *complete* keto experience, nourishing you and empowering you in every way. So I include these two 24-hour fasts because I want to provide you with a way you can fast that still gives you all the benefits of fasting without having to do a week-long hardcore fast. It's still going to be hard, but not as hard, and you'll get all the benefits.

You might be thinking, "Drew, I can't last a day without food. No way." You really can. Actually, the longest therapeutic fast in history lasted 382 days![6] It was done under medical supervision by a 27-year-old weighing 456 pounds at the start. The only things he consumed were calorie-free liquids and vitamins as monitored by health care professionals. He got down to a normal and healthy weight for him and then he maintained a healthy weight. Now, I'm not recommending this to anyone, but what I am trying to say is that you can last a long time on your own fat stores. You're not gonna die after 24 hours without food. Trust me. It will help you get into ketosis faster, it will be great for your skin and your cells, and it might even give you a big boost of confidence and clarity.

Not everybody wants to fast to get into ketosis. I get that. Know that it is optional. If it feels too intimidating you don't have to do it, you can just start with the first day of the meal plan (and then double two of the days at the end to give you a full 30 days of meals). But if you want to get into ketosis quicker and you want to explore all the other physical, mental, and spiritual benefits it offers, these two days will definitely help you out. We'll have a support system ready for you if you join the private Facebook group, where you can ask about the fast and have a community to help you get mentally prepared. That way, you'll go through it with a bunch of people where you can all share tips for surviving it and encourage and support each other through it. Join us!

So how do you fast?

I like to do the 24-hour fast on a Sunday when you (hopefully) have some downtime and can really pay attention to what you're feeling and how your body is working. Do all your grocery shopping for the week on Saturday (you'll see weekly grocery lists at the start of each week), fast on Sunday, and then start the meal plan and workouts on a Monday. Here are the approved liquids you can have—you'll be consuming only these liquids during the 24 hours of your fast:

> Water—just plain, but you can also add a whole squeezed lemon

> Electrolytes—sodium (sea salt and pink Himalayan salt are the best), magnesium, and potassium in pill form as needed. If you feel lethargic or experience brain fog while fasting, maybe do a salt shot with lots of water and a couple pills of magnesium citrate or glycinate and potassium citrate. Note that when I say electrolytes I don't mean Gatorade and Powerade—those are sugar water with a little bit of electrolytes in them. Instead, drink my electrolyte recipe.

Some of the liquids below have calories in them, which "technically" breaks a fast, but they're minimal and still have many positive effects on the body. I picked the ones that have more positive benefits than the negative of "technically" breaking a fast:

- ➤ Bone broth

- ➤ Exogenous ketones

- ➤ Apple cider vinegar—this stuff has a super strong and bitter taste, so I wouldn't go gulping it down; instead, try adding 1 or 2 tablespoons to water with a squeeze of lemon

- ➤ Powdered greens (no added sugar, mixed with water; Complete Wellness Brand is delicious in water)

- ➤ Black coffee and tea caffeinated or decaffeinated with no fats added

Before getting started, you'll definitely want to make sure you have all these liquids up and ready to go so they're there when you reach for them. I also recommend spending some time naming your why again. What's your why for doing this? Not to get all inside your head, but have it be something more than just weight loss. Fasting will get you into ketosis quicker and you'll feel the benefits sooner, not to mention the spiritual and emotional components to starting and ending your 30-day program this way. So have that why in mind so you can use it for support and encouragement during your 24-hour fast.

LET'S GET TO IT!

Okay, you're ready to get started! I'm so excited for you!

In the pages ahead you'll find 30 days of meal plans and workouts, plus checklists for affirmations and time spent in meditation. You'll see that each week starts with a grocery list and then detailed daily meal plans, which you can adjust to your taste, mixing and matching lunches and dinners, or having leftovers if you've got them. You could mix and match the breakfasts with other meals, too, but then you'd be drinking coffee at night, so I recommend following the breakfast plan for all 30 days so you keep your caffeine drinking earlier in the day and have your bigger meals at lunch and dinner. I've also included some tips and guidelines for workouts, affirmations, and meditations throughout.

If the list of things "to do" seems long, try thinking of it as an "I Get to Do This" list instead—rather than a list of things you *have* to do, flip the switch and realize that you're investing in your own physical, mental, and spiritual health. It's okay if you can't do everything, and it's okay if you feel overwhelmed some days and all you can manage is to feed yourself good, nourishing food. This shouldn't be a chore, although I know it can be very difficult, so remember to think of it in a positive way: "I get to do this" versus "I have to do this."

As you make your way through each week of the program, take a look at the week ahead to see what it looks like so you feel prepared. Each week I will be providing you shopping lists, which have everything you'll need to buy for meals that week—I recommend taking a screenshot of the list provided to take with you to the store, or you can go to fit2fat2fit.com\completeketobook to find a free downloadable grocery list to print and check off as you go.

While each week's grocery list will vary slightly from the last, there are a few staple items you'll want to have on hand for the full program. To make your transition into a ketogenic lifestyle easier, it's a great idea to start by stocking your pantry with some of these Complete Keto must-haves.

Complete Keto Must-Haves

Some things on this list, like ghee and MCT oil powder, may be hard to find at your local grocery store, so check out your local health food store, ethnic stores, or, if all else fails, online:

- ➤ Ghee

- ➤ Vanilla MCT oil powder (shop.completewellness.com)

- ➤ Avocado oil

- ➤ Coconut flour

- ➤ Apple cider vinegar

- ➤ Paleo mayo (Or make your own! See page 183 for the recipe.)

- ➤ Paleo ranch (You can also make your own—see page 184.)

- ➤ Sea salt or pink Himalayan salt

- ➤ Chili powder

- ➤ Garlic & herb seasoning blend

- ➤ Cinnamon

- ➤ Pepper

- ➤ Paprika

- ➤ Smoked paprika

- ➤ Stevia (or monkfruit, erythritol)

- ➤ Cumin

- ➤ Garlic powder

- ➤ Onion powder

- ➤ Dried parsley

- ➤ Lemon pepper

- ➤ Baking powder

- ➤ Vanilla extract

- ➤ Almond extract

One last note before we jump into the program: this is just 30 days out of your life. It can seem daunting to have to do all this—and I know you're probably feeling like you want to do it perfectly so you get it just right. So this is your reminder to be kind to yourself. This can be hard, but you can do hard things. My team and I are here to help you out and we're here to support you along the way. You're worth it to fight for your health.

WEEK ONE

The first week is all about transition—this is all still a bit new for you, and you're getting used to following a meal plan and eating keto. Your body is transitioning too, from running on glucose to producing and running on ketones. This is the period you're most likely to feel brain fog, lack of energy, and other symptoms of the keto flu. So this week really affirm your trust in the process and in yourself. You can do it!

GROCERY AND PANTRY LIST
Veg*n Approved Foods List can be found on pages 127–128

VEGETABLES	MEAT	MISC.
ASPARAGUS	BACON (1 package/12 slices)	EGGS (2 dozen)
AVOCADO (1)	BONE-IN PORK CHOP (5 ounces)	CHIPOTLE MAYO
BROCCOLI	CHICKEN APPLE SAUSAGES	COCONUT MILK (in a can)
BROCCOLINI	CHICKEN THIGHS (17 ounces)	LOW-CARB MARINARA SAUCE
CAULIFLOWER RICE (also known as cauliflower pearls)	FLANK STEAK (8 ounces)	MUSTARD
COLLARD GREENS	GROUND BEEF CHUCK (3 ounces)	OLIVE OIL
GREEN BEANS	GROUND BISON (6 ounces)	PESTO
LEMON JUICE	GROUND PORK (3 ounces)	PICKLES
MINCED GARLIC	GROUND SIRLOIN (5 ounces)	PICKLE RELISH (no sugar added)
MUSHROOMS	PORK SAUSAGE (3 ounces)	PORK RINDS
ROMAINE HEARTS	RIB EYE STEAK (6 ounces)	WHITE VINEGAR
ROMAINE SALAD MIX	SALMON FILET (6 ounces)	
SHREDDED CABBAGE		
SPINACH		
ZUCCHINI (3)		

DAY 1

(preferably Monday, after 24-hour fast Sunday)

MEAL 1	MEAL 2	MEAL 3
7 A.M.	**12 P.M.**	**6 P.M.**
Drew's Phat Coffee	Bacon Burger Salad	Grilled Rib Eye & Asparagus

DAY 1 MACROS
1,511 calories, 123g fat, 22g carbs, 81g protein (15g net carbs)

☐ POSITIVE AFFIRMATION

Living keto doesn't have to be all awesome all the time—it's an awesome program and it will change your life, for sure, but it's also a transition, and that can be hard. When you have moments or days when you're feeling doubt, craving your old habits and foods, or feeling like you've hit a plateau, you may not feel very much like doing a positive affirmation. But we aren't doing positive affirmations because everything is perfect; we're doing them to love ourselves a little more, not just when things are good but when things are hard. We're doing them so we can feel all the ups and downs of the journey without giving up or self-sabotaging.

It's normal for feelings to come up when you're making a big life change. So rather than beating yourself up, today I'm asking you to name something that challenges you—a food you've given up that you miss, a food you're eating now but don't like that much, the movement part, the meditation part, whatever—and put a positive spin on it for yourself. Maybe it's "I am brave," "I can do this," "Trust," or "My health is worth fighting for." You don't have to believe it to say it! You don't have to feel it to say it! It's powerful enough to notice what you're struggling with and then give yourself some encouragement to keep on keeping on.

Remember to speak your positive statements out loud,
possibly while looking in a mirror if you wish.

❑ MEDITATION

Aim for 5 to 10 minutes meditating. You can track how much time you were able to get in in the space provided here and throughout the rest of my plan. If you already have a regular meditation practice, please keep doing what you're doing. If you're new to meditation, try a meditation app or podcast—or just set a 10-minute alarm on your phone and give it your best shot!

Remember, in meditation your aim is to become the observer of your thoughts instead of chasing your thoughts. When thoughts come in, see them come and then watch them go. It's not about not thinking, it's about not getting all attached and reacting to those thoughts. When a thought comes in, see it as a leaf floating on a river and watch it float away downstream. Or see it as a cloud floating by.

Be in a comfortable position, wherever and however you can feel most relaxed, leaning on something if sitting up for 5 to 10 minutes is uncomfortable. Or try a walking meditation, where you spend time walking quietly in nature, paying attention to the sounds and sights around you. Remember, meditation can be done anytime, anywhere. There is no perfect time or place, so don't put pressure on yourself. Just commit to the time with no expectations!

❑ WORKOUT

AMRAP = As Many Reps As Possible. In this workout you'll be counting your TOTAL reps that you achieve in the 9 minutes that you'll be performing these three movements. So you'll have a timer in front of you and you'll perform as many burpees as you can in 1 minute. Then you'll immediately switch to sit-ups and perform as many of those as you can in 1 minute while keeping a tally of all the reps you performed (so if you finish 10 burpees in 1 minute, your first sit-up will be rep #11, and so on). Then you'll immediately switch to mountain climbers and you'll count those on top of the number of burpees and sit-ups you performed. Then you'll take a 60-second break before repeating this sequence two more times for a total of three rounds.

So let's say you did 10 burpees, 15 sit-ups, and 40 mountain climbers. Your total for round 1 would be 65 reps. In round 2 you start counting from 65 and continue. Then let's say your total after round 2 was 120. You'll start counting from 120 when you begin round 3. At the end of your workout you should have a total of number of reps performed, and that is your score for that week.

Don't be fooled, though . . . 9 minutes doesn't seem like a long time, until you do this workout. You'll be shocked at how hard a 9-minute workout can be.

ROUND 1	**ROUND 2**	**ROUND 3**
1 min. max burpees	1 min. max burpees	1 min. max burpees
1 min. max sit-ups	1 min. max sit-ups	1 min. max sit-ups
1 min. max mountain climbers	1 min. max mountain climbers	1 min. max mountain climbers
REST 1 min.	REST 1 min.	

NOTE FOR DAY 1: If you're up for testing, don't forget to test your ketones today! I recommend testing at night, because your ketones will be lower in the morning. If you do test in the morning and see a low number, don't freak out. Just know that's normal for them to be higher at night than in the morning.

DAY 2
(Tuesday)

MEAL 1

Drew's
Phat Coffee

MEAL 2

Sausage Scramble

MEAL 3

Grilled Chicken Thighs
with Sautéed Cauliflower
Medley

DAY 2 MACROS

1,443 calories, 117g fat, 22g carbs, 73g protein (18g net carbs)

🔲 POSITIVE AFFIRMATION

"I'm proud of myself."

🔲 MEDITATION

Time spent meditating: _____

🔲 WORKOUT

Timed workout! In this workout you'll be competing against the clock. You'll start the timer as soon as you start your first rep of squats and you'll let it run until you finish your last rep of step-ups. Once you complete your last step-up, you stop the clock and note your time. This time will be used next week when you repeat this workout. The goal is to beat your score week after week.

TIMED WORKOUT

100 air squats for time
100 lunges (each side) for time
100 step-ups (total) for time

Don't forget to test your ketones today!

Weekly reminder for the workouts—track your score each day. Remember to compare Week Two to Week One, Week Three to Week Two, and Week Four to Week Three, but then also Week Four to Week One, so you can see where you've come in four weeks. And if you're looking for a good pre-workout boost, do a salt shot (½ teaspoon of nutrient-dense salt) with a water chaser 20 minutes before workout. This opens blood vessels and reduces lactic acid buildup, which means less cramping!

DAY 3
(Wednesday)

MEAL 1

Drew's
Phat Coffee

MEAL 2

Bacon Avocado Egg
Salad Wraps

MEAL 3

Smoked Chili Pork Chop
with Green Beans

DAY 3 MACROS
1,427 calories, 120g fat, 23g carbs, 72g protein (16g net carbs)

📋 POSITIVE AFFIRMATION

Today I encourage you to think about what you've learned so far. What have you learned about your body? Your health? Your digestion? What have you noticed about your emotional connection to certain types of foods?

Say your answer out loud in a positive way. Maybe it's "I can do hard things," "I am stronger than my cravings," "I am open to trying new things," or "The scale doesn't define me." Whatever your answer to these questions, use it to create a positive affirmation that reflects the changes that are happening in your body from living this ketogenic lifestyle.

📋 MEDITATION

Time spent meditating: _____

📋 WORKOUT

AMRAP = As Many Reps As Possible. In this workout you're trying to complete as many reps as possible in 12 minutes. Start the timer and you'll start out each round with 30 seconds of plank immediately followed by 15 push-ups and 10 burpees. Then you start back over with 30 seconds of plank and continue this sequence until the 12 minutes is up. When the 12 minutes is up you'll tally up how many reps you completed (30-second plank doesn't count as any reps in this workout, so you'll count only the number of push-ups and burpees). Next week when you revisit this workout on Week Two, Day 10, you'll try and beat the number of reps you did the previous week.

AMRAP 12 MIN.

30-second plank
15 push-ups
10 burpees

Don't forget to test your ketones today!

DAY 4
(Thursday)

MEAL 1

Drew's
Phat Coffee

MEAL 2

BLA (Bacon, Lettuce,
Avocado) Wraps

MEAL 3

Garlic & Herb Flank Steak
with Broccoli

DAY 4 MACROS

1,475 calories, 126g fat, 23g carbs, 74g protein (14g net carbs)

☐ POSITIVE AFFIRMATION

"I am strong."

☐ MEDITATION

Time spent meditating: _____

☐ WORKOUT

In this workout you'll be holding each position for as long as you can. So you'll record your maximum time for each movement. Once you complete each movement, move quickly into the next movement and restart the timer. Take note of your time for each movement; next week when you revisit this workout the goal is to improve your time week after week.

HOLD FOR TIME

Wall sits
Side plank (each side)
Leg raise
Superman

Don't forget to test your ketones today!

DAY 5
(Friday)

MEAL 1
Drew's
Phat Coffee

MEAL 2
Chicken Pesto
Salad

MEAL 3
Bison
Bacon Burger

DAY 5 MACROS
1,443 calories, 120g fat, 19g carbs, 70g protein (14g net carbs)

☐ POSITIVE AFFIRMATION
"I am brave."

☐ MEDITATION
Time spent meditating: _____

☐ WORKOUT

AMRAP = As Many Reps As Possible. In this workout you're trying to complete as many reps as possible in 15 minutes. Start the timer and begin with 20 dips followed by 15 mountain climbers and then 10 jumping squats. Repeat this sequence, counting your total number of reps, until the 15 minutes is complete. Take note of your total number of reps performed and compare results week to week.

AMRAP 15 MIN.

20 dips
15 mountain climbers
10 jumping squats

Don't forget to test your ketones today!

DAY 6
(Saturday)

MEAL 1	**MEAL 2**	**MEAL 3**
Black coffee/fast	Chicken Apple Sausage Scramble	Lemon Pepper Salmon with Coleslaw & Asparagus

DAY 6 MACROS
1,480 calories, 118g fat, 21g carbs, 84g protein (13g net carbs)

❑ POSITIVE AFFIRMATION
"I am worthy."

❑ MEDITATION
Time spent meditating: _____

❑ WORKOUT
Enjoy a walk, yoga, or something fun with your friends or family.

Don't forget to test your ketones today!

DAY 7
(Sunday)

MEAL 1	MEAL 2	MEAL 3
Black coffee/fast	Cinnamon Pancakes with Bacon & Eggs	Zoodles & Meatballs

DAY 7 MACROS
1,516 calories, 125g fat, 13g carbs, 73g protein (8g net carbs)

❑ POSITIVE AFFIRMATION
"I love myself."

❑ MEDITATION
Time spent meditating: _____

❑ WORKOUT
Enjoy a walk, yoga, or something fun with your friends or family.

Don't forget to test your ketones today!

WEEK TWO

Hello, Week Two! By now you know that the food on keto tastes really good! During Week Two, the sun is starting to break through the clouds as your body gets more and more efficient at using ketones. But maybe you're still having moments of craving or doubt. That's normal. So rather than thinking about what you're not eating, focus on enjoying what you are eating and how it is sustaining and healing your body.

GROCERY AND PANTRY LIST*

Some items you may still have from last week.
Check to see what you still have on hand so you don't end up buying too much.

VEGETABLES	MEAT	MISC.
ASPARAGUS (2 stalks)	ANDOUILLE SAUSAGE	EGGS (18 count)
AVOCADO (2)	BACON (1 package/15 slices)	CAYENNE PEPPER
BELL PEPPER (1)	CHICKEN BREAST (8 ounces)	CHIPOTLE MAYO
BROCCOLI	CHICKEN THIGHS (2 ounces)	COCONUT AMINOS
CAULIFLOWER	FILET MIGNON (5 ounces)	COCONUT OIL
CAULIFLOWER RICE (also known as cauliflower pearls)	FLAT IRON STEAK (6 ounces)	DIJON MUSTARD
CUCUMBER (2)	GROUND BEEF (4 ounces)	GREEK VINAIGRETTE DRESSING
GUACAMOLE	GROUND PORK SAUSAGE (3 ounces)	GROUND GINGER
ICEBERG	RIB EYE STEAK (12 ounces)	KALAMATA OLIVES
MINCED GARLIC	SALMON FILET (6 ounces)	PORK RINDS
ONION (1)	SMOKED SALMON (6½ ounces)	SHREDDED UNSWEETENED COCONUT
ROMAINE HEART		
ROMAINE SALAD MIX		
SPRING SALAD MIX		
SPINACH		
TOMATO (1)		
ZUCCHINI (1)		
YELLOW SQUASH (1)		

DAY 8
(Monday)

MEAL 1	MEAL 2	MEAL 3
Drew's Phat Coffee	Keto Cobb Salad	Rib Eye Steak & Egg with Asparagus

DAY 8 MACROS
1,482 calories, 122g fat, 24g carbs, 77g protein (14g net carbs)

❏ POSITIVE AFFIRMATION
Choose your own. I've provided some examples on page 125.

❏ MEDITATION
Time spent meditating: _____

❏ WORKOUT
AMRAP = As Many Reps As Possible. In this workout you'll be counting your TOTAL reps that you achieve in the 9 minutes that you'll be performing these three movements. So you'll have a timer in front of you and you'll perform as many burpees as you can in 1 minute. Then you'll immediately switch to sit-ups and perform as many of those as you can in 1 minute while keeping a tally of all the reps you performed (so if you finish 10 burpees in 1 minute, your first sit-up will be rep #11 and so on). Then you'll immediately switch to mountain climbers and you'll count those on top of the number of burpees and sit-ups you performed. Then you'll take a 60-second break before repeating this sequence two more times for a total of three rounds.

So let's say you did 10 burpees, 15 sit-ups, and 40 mountain climbers. Your total for round 1 would be 65 reps. In round 2 you start counting from 65 and continue. Then let's say your total after round 2 was 120. You'll start counting from 120 when you begin round 3. At the end of your workout you should have a total of number of reps performed, and that is your score for that week.

Don't be fooled, though . . . 9 minutes doesn't seem like a long time, until you do this workout. You'll be shocked at how hard a 9-minute workout can be.

ROUND 1	ROUND 2	ROUND 3
1 min. max burpees	1 min. max burpees	1 min. max burpees
1 min. max sit-ups	1 min. max sit-ups	1 min. max sit-ups
1 min. max mountain climbers	1 min. max mountain climbers	1 min. max mountain climbers
REST 1 min.	REST 1 min.	

Don't forget to test your ketones today!

DAY 9
(Tuesday)

MEAL 1	MEAL 2	MEAL 3
Drew's Phat Coffee	Greek Steak Salad	Fried Chicken & Bacon Broccoli

DAY 9 MACROS
1,478 calories, 113g fat, 29g carbs, 72g protein (19g net carbs)

☐ POSITIVE AFFIRMATION
Choose your own. I've provided some examples on page 125.

☐ MEDITATION
Time spent meditating: _____

☐ WORKOUT
Timed workout! In this workout you'll be competing against the clock. You'll start the timer as soon as you start your first rep of squats and you'll let it run until you finish your last rep of step-ups. Once you complete your last step-up, you stop the clock and note your time. This time will be used next week when you repeat this workout. The goal is to beat your score week after week.

TIMED WORKOUT
100 air squats for time
100 lunges (each side) for time
100 step-ups (total) for time

Don't forget to test your ketones today!

DAY 10

(Wednesday)

MEAL 1	MEAL 2	MEAL 3
Drew's Phat Coffee	Smoked Salmon Wedge Salad	Beef & Broccoli Stir-Fry

DAY 10 MACROS

1,556 calories, 128g fat, 27g carbs, 71g protein (19g net carbs)

❏ POSITIVE AFFIRMATION

Choose your own. I've provided some examples on page 125.

❏ MEDITATION

Time spent meditating: _____

❏ WORKOUT

AMRAP = As Many Reps As Possible. In this workout you're trying to complete as many reps as possible in 12 minutes. Start the timer and you'll start out each round with 30 seconds of plank immediately followed by 15 push-ups and 10 burpees. Then you start back over with 30 seconds of plank and continue this sequence until the 12 minutes is up. When the 12 minutes is up you'll tally up how many reps you completed (30-second plank doesn't count as any reps in this workout, so you'll count only the number of push-ups and burpees). Next week when you revisit this workout on Week Three, Day 17, you'll try and beat the number of reps you did the previous week.

AMRAP 12 MIN.

30-second plank
15 push-ups
10 burpees

Don't forget to test your ketones today!

DAY 11

(Thursday)

MEAL 1	**MEAL 2**	**MEAL 3**
Drew's Phat Coffee	Drew's B.A.E.	Coconut Crusted Salmon with Spring Salad

DAY 11 MACROS

1,492 calories, 124g fat, 26g carbs, 71g protein (16g net carbs)

❑ POSITIVE AFFIRMATION

Choose your own. I've provided some examples on page 125.

❑ MEDITATION

Time spent meditating: _____

❑ WORKOUT

In this workout you'll be holding each position for as long as you can. So you'll record your maximum time for each movement. Once you complete each movement move quickly into the next movement and restart the timer. Take note of your time for each movement, and next week when you revisit this workout the goal is to improve your time week after week.

HOLD FOR TIME

Wall sits
Side plank (each side)
Leg raise
Superman

You've tested for 10 days—awesome! Now it's time to let go.
I don't recommend testing at all for the rest of the program.
For testing on keto long-term, see Part 4!

DAY 12
(Friday)

MEAL 1	**MEAL 2**	**MEAL 3**
Drew's Phat Coffee	Smoked Salmon & Poached Eggs with Hollandaise Sauce	Filet Mignon with Roasted Cauliflower

DAY 12 MACROS
1,486 calories, 124g fat, 20g carbs, 76g protein (13g net carbs)

❑ POSITIVE AFFIRMATION
Choose your own. I've provided some examples on page 125.

❑ MEDITATION
Time spent meditating: _____

❑ WORKOUT
AMRAP = As Many Reps As Possible. In this workout you're trying to complete as many reps as possible in 15 minutes. Start the timer and begin with 20 dips followed by 15 mountain climbers and then 10 jumping squats. Repeat this sequence, counting your total number of reps, until the 15 minutes is complete. Take note of your total number of reps performed and compare results week to week.

AMRAP 15 MIN.
20 dips
15 mountain climbers
10 jumping squats

DAY 13
(Saturday)

MEAL 1	MEAL 2	MEAL 3
Black coffee/fast	Savory Sausage Open-Face Sandwich	Guacamole Burger with Bacon-Wrapped Asparagus Stacks

DAY 13 MACROS
1,475 calories, 119g fat, 29g carbs, 72g protein (13g net carbs)

☐ POSITIVE AFFIRMATION
Choose your own. I've provided some examples on page 125.

☐ MEDITATION
Time spent meditating: _____

☐ WORKOUT
Enjoy a walk, yoga, or something fun with your friends or family.

DAY 14
(Sunday)

MEAL 1	MEAL 2	MEAL 3
Black coffee/fast	Dijon Mustard Chicken Salad	Smoked Sausage & Roasted Vegetables

DAY 14 MACROS
1,592 calories, 122g fat, 26g carbs, 70g protein (19g net carbs)

❏ POSITIVE AFFIRMATION
Choose your own. I've provided some examples on page 125.

❏ MEDITATION
Time spent meditating: _____

❏ WORKOUT
Enjoy a walk, yoga, or something fun with your friends or family.

WEEK THREE

You're likely to start seeing results this third week, to feel things clicking—getting into a flow with meal plans, things start working better, and your mental clarity improves. Awesome! This is keto! This week is a great time to focus on really getting in touch with your inner voice, to enjoy the changes in your body, and to cheer yourself on toward Week Four!

GROCERY AND PANTRY LIST*

*Some items you may still have from last week.
Check to see what you still have on hand so you don't end up buying too much.*

VEGETABLES	MEAT	MISC.
AVOCADO (1)	ANDOUILLE SAUSAGE	EGGS (15 count)
BABY BELLA MUSHROOMS	BACON (1 package/16 slices)	ARTICHOKE HEARTS
BELL PEPPER (2)	CHICKEN BREAST (3 ounces)	BLACK OLIVES
BROCCOLI	CHICKEN THIGHS (14 ounces)	BUFFALO SAUCE
CAULIFLOWER	CHICKEN WINGS (6 ounces)	CAESAR DRESSING (PALEO)
CAULIFLOWER RICE (also known as cauliflower pearls)	GROUND BEEF CHUCK (3 ounces)	CAJUN SEASONING
CELERY	GROUND PORK SAUSAGE (7 ounces)	CAPERS
COLLARD GREENS	POLISH SAUSAGE LINKS	CHIPOTLE SEASONING
GREEN ONIONS (also known as spring onions)	PORK BREAKFAST SAUSAGE (3 ounces)	COCONUT AMINOS
GUACAMOLE	RIB EYE STEAK (4 ounces)	GREEK VINAIGRETTE DRESSING
LEMON (1)	SALMON FILLET (4 ounces)	GROUND GINGER
MINCED GARLIC	SHREDDED ROAST BEEF (4 ounces)	HEMP HEARTS
ONION (1)		HOT SAUCE
ROMAINE HEART		ITALIAN SEASONING
RADISHES		LOW-CARB MARINARA
SHREDDED CABBAGE		MUSTARD
SLICED MUSHROOMS		OREGANO
SPRING SALAD MIX		RED WINE VINEGAR
SPINACH		RED PEPPER FLAKES
THYME		SESAME OIL
TOMATO (1)		THYME
ZUCCHINI (2)		WHITE WINE VINEGAR

MEAL 1	**MEAL 2**	**MEAL 3**
Drew's Phat Coffee	Steak & Eggs Breakfast Scramble	Buffalo Wings & Coleslaw

DAY 15 MACROS
1,522 calories, 127g fat, 22g carbs, 73g protein (18g net carbs)

❏ POSITIVE AFFIRMATION

Choose your own. I've provided some examples on page 125.

❏ MEDITATION

Time spent meditating: _____

❏ WORKOUT

AMRAP = As Many Reps As Possible. In this workout you'll be counting your TOTAL reps that you achieve in the 9 minutes that you'll be performing these three movements. So you'll have a timer in front of you and you'll perform as many burpees as you can in 1 minute. Then you'll immediately switch to sit-ups and perform as many of those as you can in 1 minute while keeping a tally of all the reps you performed (so if you finish 10 burpees in 1 minute, your first sit-up will be rep #11 and so on). Then you'll immediately switch to mountain climbers and you'll count those on top of the number of burpees and sit-ups you performed. Then you'll take a 60-second break before repeating this sequence two more times for a total of three rounds.

So let's say you did 10 burpees, 15 sit-ups, and 40 mountain climbers. Your total for round 1 would be 65 reps. In round 2 you start counting from 65 and continue. Then let's say your total after round 2 was 120. You'll start counting from 120 when you begin round 3. At the end of your workout you should have a total of number of reps performed, and that is your score for that week.

Don't be fooled, though . . . 9 minutes doesn't seem like a long time, until you do this workout. You'll be shocked at how hard a 9-minute workout can be.

ROUND 1
1 min. max burpees
1 min. max sit-ups
1 min. max mountain climbers
REST 1 min.

DAY 16
(Tuesday)

MEAL 1	**MEAL 2**	**MEAL 3**
Drew's Phat Coffee	Taco Salad & Chipotle Dressing	Polish Sausage with Fried Cabbage & Collard Greens

DAY 16 MACROS
1,495 calories, 127g fat, 28g carbs, 64g protein (21g net carbs)

☐ POSITIVE AFFIRMATION

Choose your own. I've provided some examples on page 125.

☐ MEDITATION

Time spent meditating: _____

☐ WORKOUT

Timed workout! In this workout you'll be competing against the clock. You'll start the timer as soon as you start your first rep of squats and you'll let it run until you finish your last rep of step-ups. Once you complete your last step-up, you stop the clock and note your time. This time will be used next week when you repeat this workout. The goal is to beat your score week after week.

TIMED WORKOUT
100 air squats
100 lunges (each side)
100 step-ups (total)

DAY 17
(Wednesday)

MEAL 1
Drew's
Phat Coffee

MEAL 2
Bacon Veggie
Omelette

MEAL 3
Chicken Artichoke
Zoodle Pan

DAY 17 MACROS
1,477 calories, 121g fat, 26g carbs, 72g protein (19g net carbs)

❏ POSITIVE AFFIRMATION
Choose your own. I've provided some examples on page 125.

❏ MEDITATION
Time spent meditating: _____

❏ WORKOUT
AMRAP = As Many Reps As Possible. In this workout you're trying to complete as many reps as possible in 12 minutes. Start the timer and you'll start out each round with 30 seconds of plank immediately followed by 15 push-ups and 10 burpees. Then you start back over with 30 seconds of plank and continue this sequence until the 12 minutes is up. When the 12 minutes is up you'll tally up how many reps you completed (30-second plank doesn't count as any reps in this workout, so you'll count only the number of push-ups and burpees). Next week when you revisit this workout on Week Four, Day 24, you'll try and beat the number of reps you did the previous week.

AMRAP 12 MIN.
30-second plank
15 push-ups
10 burpees

DAY 18
(Thursday)

MEAL 1	MEAL 2	MEAL 3
Drew's Phat Coffee	Chicken Club Wraps	Keto Chicken Chow Mein

DAY 18 MACROS
1,478 calories, 122g fat, 27g carbs, 68g protein (18g net carbs)

☐ POSITIVE AFFIRMATION
Choose your own. I've provided some examples on page 125.

☐ MEDITATION
Time spent meditating: _____

☐ WORKOUT
In this workout you'll be holding each position for as long as you can. So you'll record your maximum time for each movement. Once you complete each movement, move quickly into the next movement and restart the timer. Take note of your time for each movement, and next week when you revisit this workout the goal is to improve your time week after week.

HOLD FOR TIME
Wall sits
Side plank (each side)
Leg raise
Superman

DAY 19
(Friday)

MEAL 1	**MEAL 2**	**MEAL 3**
Drew's Phat Coffee	Sausage Frittata & Fried Radishes	Unstuffed Peppers

DAY 19 MACROS
1,501 calories, 125g fat, 28g carbs, 66g protein (20g net carbs)

❏ POSITIVE AFFIRMATION
Choose your own. I've provided some examples on page 125.

❏ MEDITATION
Time spent meditating: _____

❏ WORKOUT

AMRAP = As Many Reps As Possible. In this workout you're trying to complete as many reps as possible in 15 minutes. Start the timer and begin with 20 dips followed by 15 mountain climbers and then 10 jumping squats. Repeat this sequence, counting your total number of reps, until the 15 minutes is complete. Take note of your total number of reps performed and compare results week to week.

AMRAP 15 MIN.
20 dips
15 mountain climbers
10 jumping squats

DAY 20
(Saturday)

MEAL 1	MEAL 2	MEAL 3
Black coffee/fast	Keto-rito	Jambalaya

DAY 20 MACROS
1,494 calories, 121g fat, 24g carbs, 77g protein (16g net carbs)

☐ POSITIVE AFFIRMATION
Choose your own. I've provided some examples on page 125.

☐ MEDITATION
Time spent meditating: _____

☐ WORKOUT
Enjoy a walk, yoga, or something fun with your friends or family.

DAY 21
(Sunday)

MEAL 1	MEAL 2	MEAL 3
Black coffee/fast	Caesar Chicken Salad	Bacon-Wrapped Salmon

DAY 21 MACROS

1,523 calories, 124g fat, 16g carbs, 76g protein (9g net carbs)

❑ POSITIVE AFFIRMATION
Choose your own. I've provided some examples on page 125.

❑ MEDITATION
Time spent meditating: _____

❑ WORKOUT
Enjoy a walk, yoga, or something fun with your friends or family.

HOW TO HANDLE PLATEAUS

You've been following the meal plans. You're feeling great. You've seen some initial success and things are going well. But what if you hit Day 23 and realize you haven't seen progress in the past few days. What do you do? So many people come to me asking how to overcome a plateau because they haven't seen any progress in the past few days even though they're doing everything they're supposed to. First of all, I can totally relate.

When I did my Fit2Fat2Fit journey there were a couple weeks where I gained weight and didn't lose any. Here I was, a personal trainer with all the knowledge and discipline a person could have, and I was eating what I was supposed to and exercising like how I was supposed to, but I wasn't losing weight.

What I learned is that I was focusing too much on weight loss and the number on the scale, rather than enjoying the journey. A plateau can exist only if you're focusing on the end goal more than the process. So if you feel you're hitting a plateau, here are a few reminders:

➤ What's your definition of a plateau? If you're just basing it on weight loss, then most likely you're not hitting a plateau—weight loss is not linear, it's not black and white. There are lots of variables.

➤ Make sure you take measurements or get your body fat tested—those are better ways to measure progress than the scale. If you're seeing progress on your work-outs week to week, you're not hitting a plateau—your body is changing!

➤ The goal isn't weight loss, it's fat loss, and the only way to measure that is to get your body tested. The scale can't measure that.

➤ Focus on the process and not the results. This isn't a race to some imaginary finish line. This is a lifestyle change. If you just focus on the results, you'll get tired of the process. Focus on the process and the results will take care of themselves.

➤ There's more to weight loss than just being skinny—being healthy actually has more to do with loving yourself. Don't forget to do your meditations and positive affirmations so you give yourself a good dose of self-love today!

Healing isn't always a straight line—it takes ups and downs, and stops and starts. So if today you feel frustrated because you're not seeing the results you'd like to see, take a deep breath and allow yourself to just be where you are. No plateaus, no disappointment, or seeking the finish line. Just appreciate yourself for every healthy habit you do.

WEEK FOUR

You made it to Week Four! By now you're probably feeling lots of excitement—your body's changing, you're feeling stronger, and your cravings are most likely gone. This is usually the time in the program where people are feeling so good they're ready to spread the word about how amazing keto is!** So go ahead and let your affirmations, meditations, and workouts this week reflect your newly found energy, strength, confidence, and desire for connection.

GROCERY AND PANTRY LIST*

*Some items you may still have from last week.
Check to see what you still have on hand so you don't end up buying too much.*

VEGETABLES	MEAT	MISC.
ASPARAGUS (1)	BACON (1 package/14 slices)	EGGS (24 count)
AVOCADO (2)	BONE-IN PORK CHOP (6 ounces)	ALLSPICE
BELL PEPPER (2)	BEEF TOP ROUND STEAK (6 ounces)	CASHEW MILK
BUTTON MUSHROOMS	BREAKFAST SAUSAGE LINKS	CAYENNE PEPPER
BROCCOLI	CHICKEN DRUMSTICKS (4 ounces)	CHIA SEEDS
CAULIFLOWER	CHICKEN THIGHS (4 ounces)	COCONUT MILK (canned)
CHERRY TOMATOES	DICED HAM	COCONUT OIL
GREEN BEANS	FLANK STEAK (6 ounces)	CHIPOTLE SEASONING
GREEN ONIONS (also known as spring onions)	GROUND PORK BREAKFAST SAUSAGE (3 ounces)	COCONUT AMINOS
GUACAMOLE	GROUND SIRLOIN PATTY (⅓ pound)	DIJON MUSTARD
ICEBERG LETTUCE	PORK BABY BACK RIBS (5 ounces)	GARLIC OLIVE OIL
MINCED GARLIC	PULLED PORK BUTT (3 ounces)	GROUND GINGER
ONION (1)	SALMON FILLET (7 ounces)	HOT SAUCE
PICO DE GALLO		INSTANT COFFEE
PORTOBELLO MUSHROOM CAP (2)		ITALIAN SEASONING
RADISHES		LEMON JUICE
SEAFOOD HERB BLEND		NUTMEG
SLICED MUSHROOMS		PORK RINDS
SPRING SALAD MIX		RED PEPPER FLAKES
SPINACH		SHREDDED UNSWEETENED COCONUT
THYME		TACO SEASONING (no sugar added)
ZUCCHINI (2)		THYME
YELLOW SQUASH (1)		WHIPPED COCONUT CREAM

** If you don't feel this way, it's okay. For some people it just takes a little longer to let their cravings subside and to become fat-adapted. Don't give up! You'll get there, I promise. You're still doing great.

DAY 22
(Monday)

MEAL 1	MEAL 2	MEAL 3
Drew's Phat Coffee	Meat Lovers' Scramble	Jerk Chicken & Veggie Kabobs

DAY 22 MACROS
1,503 calories, 125g fat, 20g carbs, 73g protein (16g net carbs)

☐ POSITIVE AFFIRMATION
Choose your own. I've provided some examples on page 125.

☐ MEDITATION
Time spent meditating: _____

☐ WORKOUT
AMRAP = As Many Reps As Possible. In this workout you'll be counting your TOTAL reps that you achieve in the 9 minutes that you'll be performing these three movements. So you'll have a timer in front of you and you'll perform as many burpees as you can in 1 minute. Then you'll immediately switch to sit-ups and perform as many of those as you can in 1 minute while keeping a tally of all the reps you performed (so if you finish 10 burpees in 1 minute, your first sit-up will be rep #11 and so on). Then you'll immediately switch to mountain climbers and you'll count those on top of the number of burpees and sit-ups you performed. Then you'll take a 60-second break before repeating this sequence two more times for a total of three rounds.

So let's say you did 10 burpees, 15 sit-ups, and 40 mountain climbers. Your total for round 1 would be 65 reps. In round 2 you start counting from 65 and continue. Then let's say your total after round 2 was 120. You'll start counting from 120 when you begin round 3. At the end of your workout you should have a total of number of reps performed, and that is your score for that week.

Don't be fooled, though . . . 9 minutes doesn't seem like a long time, until you do this workout. You'll be shocked at how hard a 9-minute workout can be.

ROUND 1	ROUND 2	ROUND 3
1 min. max burpees	1 min. max burpees	1 min. max burpees
1 min. max sit-ups	1 min. max sit-ups	1 min. max sit-ups
1 min. max mountain climbers	1 min. max mountain climbers	1 min. max mountain climbers
REST 1 min.	REST 1 min.	

DAY 23
(Tuesday)

MEAL 1
Drew's
Phat Coffee

MEAL 2
Shredded Pork
Salad

MEAL 3
Creamy Salmon
Fillet

DAY 23 MACROS
1,471 calories, 126g fat, 24g carbs, 65g protein (15g net carbs)

❏ POSITIVE AFFIRMATION
Choose your own. I've provided some examples on page 125.

❏ MEDITATION
Time spent meditating: _____

❏ WORKOUT
Timed workout! In this workout you'll be competing against the clock. You'll start the timer as soon as you start your first rep of squats and you'll let it run until you finish your last rep of step-ups. Once you complete your last step-up, you stop the clock and note your time. This time will be used next week when you repeat this workout. The goal is to beat your score week after week.

TIMED WORKOUT
100 air squats for time
100 lunges (each side) for time
100 step-ups (total) for time

DAY 24
(Wednesday)

MEAL 1	MEAL 2	MEAL 3
Drew's Phat Coffee	English Breakfast Plate	Chipotle Portobello Mushroom Burger

DAY 24 MACROS
1,494 calories, 126g fat, 30g carbs, 65g protein (20g net carbs)

❏ POSITIVE AFFIRMATION
Choose your own. I've provided some examples on page 125.

❏ MEDITATION
Time spent meditating: _____

❏ WORKOUT
AMRAP = As Many Reps As Possible. In this workout you're trying to complete as many reps as possible in 12 minutes. Start the timer and you'll start out each round with 30 seconds of plank immediately followed by 15 push-ups and 10 burpees. Then you start back over with 30 seconds of plank and continue this sequence until the 12 minutes is up. When the 12 minutes is up you'll tally up how many reps you completed (30-second plank doesn't count as any reps in this workout, so you'll count only the number of push-ups and burpees).

AMRAP 12 MIN.
30-second plank
15 push-ups
10 burpees

DAY 25
(Thursday)

MEAL 1	**MEAL 2**	**MEAL 3**
Drew's Phat Coffee	Avocado Egg Boats	Beef Top Round Steak with Garlic Cauliflower Mash

DAY 25 MACROS
1,443 calories, 119g fat, 25g carbs, 75g protein (14g net carbs)

☐ POSITIVE AFFIRMATION
Choose your own. I've provided some examples on page 125.

☐ MEDITATION
Time spent meditating: _____

☐ WORKOUT
In this workout you'll be holding each position for as long as you can. So you'll record your maximum time for each movement. Once you complete each movement, move quickly into the next movement and restart the timer. Take note of your time for each movement, and next week when you revisit this workout. The goal is to improve your time week after week.

HOLD FOR TIME
Wall sits
Side plank
Leg raise
Superman

DAY 26
(Friday)

MEAL 1	MEAL 2	MEAL 3
Drew's Phat Coffee	Steak Fajita Salad	Dry Rub Ribs & Lemon Garlic Roasted Vegetables

DAY 26 MACROS
1,503 calories, 124g fat, 29g carbs, 70g protein (22g net carbs)

❏ POSITIVE AFFIRMATION
Choose your own. I've provided some examples on page 125.

❏ MEDITATION
Time spent meditating: _____

❏ WORKOUT
AMRAP = As Many Reps As Possible. In this workout you're trying to complete as many reps as possible in 15 minutes. Start the timer and begin with 20 dips followed by 15 mountain climbers and then 10 jumping squats. Repeat this sequence, counting your total number of reps, until the 15 minutes is complete. Take note of your total number of reps performed and compare results week to week.

AMRAP 15 MIN.
20 dips
15 mountain climbers
10 jumping squats

DAY 27
(Saturday)

MEAL 1
Black coffee/fast

MEAL 2
Savory Waffles
with Eggs & Pico

MEAL 3
Bacon-Wrapped Chicken
Drumsticks & Fried
Zucchini

DAY 27 MACROS
1,503 calories, 127g fat, 22g carbs, 75g protein (12g net carbs)

❏ POSITIVE AFFIRMATION
Choose your own. I've provided some examples on page 125.

❏ MEDITATION
Time spent meditating: _____

❏ WORKOUT
Enjoy a walk, yoga, or something fun with your friends or family.

DAY 28

(Sunday)

MEAL 1	**MEAL 2**	**MEAL 3**
Black coffee/fast	Lemon Chia Pancakes	Baked Ranch Pork Chops with Bacon Broccoli

DAY 28 MACROS
1,509 calories, 121g fat, 28g carbs, 78g protein (19g net carbs)

☐ POSITIVE AFFIRMATION

Choose your own. I've provided some examples on page 125.

☐ MEDITATION

Time spent meditating: _____

☐ WORKOUT

Enjoy a walk, yoga, or something fun with your friends or family.

POSITIVE AFFIRMATIONS

If you get stuck coming up with your own personal affirmations, here are some bonus affirmations you can try on for size:

- "I'm proud of who I am."
- "I am happy."
- "I am healthy."
- "I am strong."
- "I can do hard things."
- "I'm worth it."
- "I nourish my body with healing food."
- "I enjoy the smell, color, and taste of my food."

- "I am nourished."
- "I'm enjoying the journey."
- "I'm proud of every step I take to improve my life and my health."
- "My mind is clear and calm."
- "I love my body."
- "I feel good and I want others to feel good, too."
- "I am strong."
- "I love enjoying life!"

VEGAN AND VEGETARIAN MEAL PLANS

Hey, veg*n friends! I know, I know. That section above is super meat heavy. But have no fear! You are very welcome here—yes, you can do plant-based keto and receive all the same anti-inflammatory, brain and energy boosting benefits.

Plant-based keto is more restrictive when it comes to food choices than my omnivore plan, but you knew that already, didn't you? Because vegetarian and vegan diets are by nature more restrictive! I do get questions from people wanting to try keto and go veg all at once, but I wouldn't try to go veg just to do keto. If you're already vegan for health, ethical, or environmental reasons, though, I'm here for you!

I remember talking with someone who told me they were very curious about keto for the health benefits but that it seemed like something only meat-eaters could do. All those photos of bacon-wrapped steak were not at all enticing for them! So I dug into some research on plant-based keto, and most of what I saw was experts saying it's too difficult to do. Um, yeah, of course it's difficult if no one's out here supporting you! I know lots of vegans and vegetarians, and they have chosen a more restrictive diet on purpose because of the things they care about, so why should they be left out of all the keto benefits just because their food selection is more limited without meat as an option? That's why I've included guidance and recipes for my plant-based friends. My veg keto meals are delicious, filling, and great for you, and tested by real-life plant-based people!

Plant-based diets tend to be high in carbohydrates because rice and beans are affordable sources of protein that can be made into all sorts of delicious meals. But veg*n keto flips the dreaded "but where do you get your protein?" question on its head, because what you want is lots of healthy fats, not a ton of protein. So instead of carb-heavy rice and beans, we're talking avocados, olives, coconut, soy, seeds, and, yes, nuts and nut butter. Shhh, don't tell the others, but my vegan keto program does allow for nuts as long as they aren't roasted in inflammatory oils.

For both vegans and vegetarians, remember that your carb macros will be slightly different from the omnivore plan—40 net carbs a day—but protein and fat are the same: 50 to 70 grams protein and 150 grams fat. Since there is no dairy on my plan, that will be the same for vegans and vegetarians, but vegetarians can do eggs as well, and fish, too, if you do fish.

A few important notes: Make sure you're eating enough! With the additional restrictions on veg*n keto, you may find yourself needing to eat more throughout the day, and that's fine. It's okay to add another meal, more snacks, or double a recipe. I recommend supplementing with a good vegan B_{12} and vitamin D_3. Feel free to add in a good-quality multivitamin, DHA, and probiotics/prebiotics as well. You may also supplement protein with a good-quality vegan protein powder.

Below you'll find a sample meal plan for seven days for vegan keto to get you started. If you're vegetarian, feel free to add eggs (and fish if you eat fish) as you like. There are lots of additional veg-friendly recipes in the recipe section, and I know you're all very good at veganizing recipes, so do your thing! I hope you'll follow along with the affirmations, meditations, and workouts in the program above too.

VEG*N APPROVED FOODS LIST

PROTEIN	FATS	NUTS
TOFU	COCONUT OIL	ALMONDS
TEMPEH	COCONUT	CASHEWS
SEITAN	ALMOND BUTTER	CHIA SEEDS
LOW-CARB VEGAN PROTEIN POWDER	PEANUT BUTTER	HAZELNUTS
	MACADAMIA NUT BUTTER	MACADAMIA NUTS
	AVOCADOS	PECANS
	AVOCADO OIL	PILI
	OLIVE OIL	PUMPKIN SEEDS
	CACAO BUTTER	SESAME SEEDS
	BUTTER (vegetarian)	SUNFLOWER SEEDS
	GHEE (vegetarian)	WALNUTS
	CHEESE (vegetarian)	CHIA SEEDS
		FLAXSEEDS

VEGETABLES	FRUITS	BAKING
ARTICHOKES	BLACKBERRIES	ALMOND FLOUR
ASPARAGUS	BLUEBERRIES	COCONUT FLOUR
BOK CHOY	RASPBERRIES	FLAXSEED MEAL
BRUSSELS SPROUTS	STRAWBERRIES	PSYLLIUM HUSK
CABBAGE		ARROWROOT POWDER
CAULIFLOWER		GUAR GUM
CELERY		ANY UNSWEETENED NONDAIRY MILK
CUCUMBER		MONK FRUIT SWEETENER
EDAMAME		STEVIA
EGGPLANT		ERYTHRITOL
GARLIC		
GREEN BEANS		
KALE		
LETTUCE		
MUSHROOMS		
PEPPERS		
RADISH		
SPINACH		
ZUCCHINI		

DAY 1

MEAL 1

Drew's Phat Coffee
(to keep it vegan, replace ghee with coconut oil or coconut cream)

MEAL 2

Berry Breakfast Bowl

MEAL 3

Broccoli Stir Fry

NUTRITION INFORMATION FOR THE DAY
1,486 calories, 120g fat, 56g carbs, 52g protein (31g net carbs)

DAY 2

MEAL 1

Drew's Phat Coffee

MEAL 2

Chocolate Strawberry Protein Smoothie

MEAL 3

Zucchini Pesto

NUTRITION INFORMATION FOR THE DAY
1,549 calories, 133g fat, 39g carbs, 56g protein (23g net carbs)

DAY 3

MEAL 1

Drew's Phat Coffee

MEAL 2

Greek Salad

MEAL 3

Spring Roll Bowl

NUTRITION INFORMATION FOR THE DAY
1,548 calories, 128g fat, 52g carbs, 42g protein (42g net carbs)

DAY 4

MEAL 1

Drew's Phat Coffee

MEAL 2

Chocolate Peanut Butter Shake

MEAL 3

Creamy Broccoli Soup

NUTRITION INFORMATION FOR THE DAY

1,452 calories, 114g fat, 62g carbs, 59g protein (33g net carbs)

DAY 5

MEAL 1

Drew's Phat Coffee

MEAL 2

Portobello Mushroom Salad with Poppy Seed Dressing

MEAL 3

Pad Thai

NUTRITION INFORMATION FOR THE DAY

1,453 calories, 123g fat, 56g carbs, 39g protein (36g carbs)

DAY 6

MEAL 1

Black coffee/fast

MEAL 2

Peanut Butter No Oats Oatmeal

MEAL 3

Zucchini Sage Pasta

NUTRITION INFORMATION FOR THE DAY

1,526 calories, 127g fat, 43g carbs, 63g protein (26g net carbs)

DAY 7

MEAL 1

Black coffee/fast

MEAL 2

Berry Protein Shake

MEAL 3

Broccoli Slaw Salad

NUTRITION INFORMATION FOR THE DAY

1,473 calories, 121g fat, 58g carbs, 49g protein (33g net carbs)

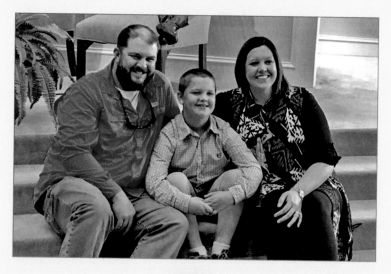

BEFORE

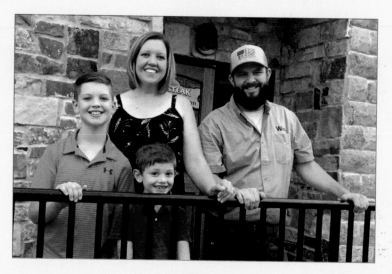

AFTER

THE KIRKMAN FAMILY

MY FAMILY & I STARTED OUR FIT2FAT2FIT JOURNEY THE FIRST WEEK OF FEBRUARY 2018. My husband and I both weighed 262, our heaviest ever! Our nine-year-old son, Zack, weighed 115 and was going down a very unhealthy path. We were all in desperate need of an intervention. We came across Drew Manning's program and felt compelled to give it a try. Drew literally put himself in our shoes, laced them up, and showed us how to get the weight off. We decided to order the eight-week program and fully committed to it. Drew's program is designed to be very easy to follow and really took the guessing game out of what you can and cannot eat. I loved the simplicity of the program and how we could follow it, even with our busy schedules. Within the first week we could already tell a huge difference in the way we were feeling. We weren't crashing on the couch in the afternoons because we were so tired. After we hit the eight-week mark, my husband and I had each lost over 20 pounds! Our son had dropped 10 pounds and we all felt amazing. We were so proud of ourselves and loving the keto lifestyle that we stuck with it and kept pressing forward. To date I have lost 60 pounds and went from a size 22/24 to a 14/16. My husband has lost 55 pounds and went from a size 38 pant to a size 36 and went from an XXL shirt to a large. Our son has lost 26 pounds and went from a boys' 14/16 to an 8/10. We have not only lost weight, we have also gained our confidence back. We have more energy than ever! Our family is healthy, happy, and thriving like never before!! We will forever be grateful to Drew and his program for changing our lives!

Many thanks,

— COURTNEY, JERRY & ZACK KIRKMAN

PART 4

PHASE TWO: KETO FOR LIFE

You just finished the CK30! Congratulations! Where do you go from here? Well, we're not done yet—like those late-night infomercials love to say, but wait, there's more!

I know it can be hard to know what to do after 30 days; I've been holding your hand and telling you what to eat every day, and how to work out every day, and after the 30 days is over it can feel like, okay, where do I go from here?

Drew, tell me what to do! As scary as it might have felt to take on 30 days of Complete Keto, it can feel even more overwhelming to be set loose on your own, especially if you're feeling great and don't want to stop feeling great (but at the same time maybe you are starting to miss going out for ice cream with your kids)!

It reminds me of the year my oldest daughter was learning to ride a bike. I admit I was a mess. It was my job to protect her and keep her safe, right? Yet here she was, excited and ready to get on what now seemed to me to be a two-wheeled death trap and ride on down the sidewalk away from me at top speed. As much as I wanted to wrap her up in protective padding and keep her safe from everything the world might bring, I also realized how ridiculous that was. I didn't want to keep her from life, I wanted to raise a strong daughter who could take care of herself. A girl who would grow into a woman with the resiliency to forge her own path and the strength to trust her own voice. Strong father, strong daughter. And that meant I couldn't hold on to the back of that bike forever. I was going to have to teach her everything I knew, take the training wheels off, and then stand back and let her learn to find her own balance and test her own boundaries, even if that meant a few falls and scraped knees.

Do you see where I'm going with this?

This book is called *Complete Keto* because it isn't just a 30-day diet plan—my goal has never been for you to just lose X amount of weight and then that's it. There is no summit, there is no finish line. It's all your life. I want to help you love the journey, because that's where life happens! And that means you need support and guidance for more than 30 days only. But just like my kid who had to go out and learn how to find her balance on that bike, and I had to let her struggle to figure it out for herself, this next phase of Complete Keto is all about taking off the training wheels and you finding the best path forward for *you*. You can't have someone there holding your hand the rest of your life, much as you may want that in this moment, and you can't have somebody telling you what to eat and how to work out every minute of every day; you have to learn and grow and figure out your own keto for life.

My hope is that you've learned all the skills you need to continue what I've given you in the past 30 days to take the reins and steer your own course. To make keto a lifestyle, not a diet. Like Chris, who wrote me that at first he wasn't sure what to expect with my program, but figured he'd try it for 60 days and see how it was going. A year later, he's still going strong on keto, no longer craves the unhealthy junk food he

used to live on, and feels better than ever. "This is only the beginning," he told me. Or Morgan, who says he's now "Keto4Life" and that the best is yet to come because he feels better about himself than he has in years. Or Patty, who told me she can't wait to see what the next months and years will bring because keto has changed her life in so many awesome ways in just three short months. Like these amazing people and so many others like them, you can make keto fit into your lifestyle and you can keep seeing great results over time!

You've got a ton of great recipes, a baseline guide for your macros and micronutrients, tips for intermittent fasting, great workouts to build from, and a practice of meditation and positive affirmations to fuel your spiritual and emotional health. As you embark now on the rest of your life, maybe ask yourself some questions about what worked and didn't work for you over the past 30 days: What foods did you love? What fun keto recipes are you inspired to look up or invent yourself? What did you learn about the power of meditation or moving your body every day? What have you learned about yourself—your body, what makes you happy, your goals in life, your why?

Have you ever seen a baby bird learn how to fly? No apparent anxiety there, just a mama bird nudging her baby out and letting instinct kick in. I promise I'm not going to go all mama bird on you and just throw you out of the nest—it's not like see you later, peace out, thanks for stopping by for 30 days. If you know exactly how you want to continue on from this 30 days, then get on that bike and ride! You don't need my permission (or if you feel you do need my permission, permission granted!). But if you're looking for guidance on where to go next, I've got you. This section includes different paths you can choose going forward based on your experience with the 30 days, like those Choose Your Own Adventure books I remember from my grade school days. If you want to commit to keto after the 30-day program, I've given protocols for three adventures you can choose from: the Targeted Keto Diet, the Cyclical Keto Diet, and the Intermittent Keto Diet.

The Targeted Keto Diet is sometimes called a "carb timing" approach, where you time your carbohydrate consumption pre- and post-workout so you're more efficient at high-intensity workouts. You'll get more out of your workouts this way. Your body is now fat-adapted, but it can still use glucose as a fuel source, so your ability to switch over from glucose to ketones should be heightened at this point. This makes the Targeted Keto Diet a good approach for those who want the ability to use both glucose and ketones as a kind of dual fuel for better performance and to maximize your workouts. It's great for athletes, especially those who do high-intensity workouts, and for those wanting more out of their workouts because they want to lose more fat or get faster. The idea is specifically timing carbohydrate intake with workouts to optimize performance and results.

The Cyclical Keto Diet is more of a maintenance phase once you become fat-adapted from the 30 days. It allows you to stay in a state of ketosis Monday through Friday, or Monday through Saturday, then you have one to two high-carb, low-fat days, and then you go right back into the keto lifestyle (and ketosis) the next day. On Cyclical Keto, your fat and carbs teeter-totter—when your carb intake goes up, your fat intake goes down, and vice versa—while your protein stays about the same.

This approach doesn't work well for people who aren't yet fat-adapted, and that's why it's important to do the 30 days of strict keto before you jump into this. Otherwise you'll never really reach the peak of being efficient at using ketones as an energy source and the back-and-forth from glucose to ketones will not work very well. But if you are fat-adapted because you've done keto for 30 (or for some people, 90) days, this is a great, balanced approach where you do keto the majority of the time, maybe 80 percent of the time, and then you have one or two days of higher carb, lower fat days.

The Intermittent Keto Diet is an approach that uses my 30-day program anywhere from one to four times a year as a cleanse or detox to reset your body. This is a good protocol for those who may want to go back to eating more of a paleo diet or a higher carb vegan or vegetarian diet most of the time, but who saw good results from the 30 days and want to do a good cleanse or detox a few times a year.

I've used all these approaches at various times for different reasons. When I'm training for a specific athletic performance like a triathlon or CrossFit competition, I will do more of the Targeted Keto Diet. I use Cyclical Keto for maintaining when I don't have any specific fitness goals and I want to maintain without missing out on having a pancake breakfast with my daughters on the weekend. Intermittent Keto I do every once in a while if I feel I want a hardcore reset in my body; I'll go more paleo for 30 to 60 days, where I include potatoes and sweet potatoes, carrots, and fruits into my diet, and then once or twice a year I do a keto cleanse.

I like to find what works best for me at any given time and then commit. I'm not an all one thing all the time type of person. We need variety to keep life interesting! Plus, our goals change over time, and so do our bodies. So think of this post-keto detox phase as a time to find what protocol works best for you. It all depends on your goals, how your body feels while eating keto, and how keto can best work with your lifestyle. Do you want to increase your performance in the gym or on race day? Do you want to maintain what you achieved during the keto detox while also finding balance so that you can enjoy birthday cake or sweet potatoes from time to time? Are you doing keto for therapeutic health purposes? Do you have a healthy lifestyle that works for you but just want a reset a couple times a year?

Now more than ever, I encourage you to be a self-experimenter. You did an awesome thing for your body, mind, and spirit by doing my 30-day keto cleanse; now it's time to experiment a little and figure out what works best for you long-term so you can love your life!

Maybe once you read more about the protocols below, none of the approaches will seem to fit in with your goals—if you feel fine with staying strict on keto and don't want to eat carbs ever again, that's fine, that's totally your choice. It's up to you. You don't have to do Targeted Keto or Cyclical Keto or ever introduce carbs back into your life. Some people feel fantastic on keto and then they try Cyclical Keto and they feel awful after eating some carb that they haven't had in a long time. And it's like, man, I don't like that feeling—I like feeling that high of mental clarity, improvement in cognitive function, not being so hungry throughout the day, and more. That's really powerful for a lot of people. Think of this post-detox time as an opportunity to experiment a little and figure out what you really want out of keto. It may take some time and a little trial and error, but remember that you and your health are worth it.

If you do find that staying 100 percent keto is what works for you, don't panic. Remember that for most people it is healthy to stay in a state of ketosis long-term. I know doctors who have done strict keto for decades, and I know people with epilepsy who have done it for years, and they're totally healthy. So if you felt amazing on keto during the 30 days and want to stay 100 percent because you learned that carbs just don't work for you anymore, or for a specific therapeutic health reason, like Parkinson's, epilepsy, or certain forms of cancer, or because your doctor advised you to, that's fine. For some people, that's the way to go.

But in my opinion, you don't have to stay strict keto for the rest of your life. There's no rule that says if you felt great on keto that you need to stay 100 percent keto. If you do, you'll be okay, but you don't have to.

Remember that our ancestors very likely dipped in and out of ketosis as part of the normal ebb and flow of their lives and the availability of food. They went through periods of feast or famine and they probably went in and out of ketosis based on their surroundings, their environment, and what types of foods were available. Maybe in the colder months there was little to no green growing things to eat, so they ate mostly meat because that's what they had and could survive on. Then in the warmer months and in times when meat was scarce, they lived off of berries and other growing edible foods they could find.

So you don't need to stay in a state of ketosis forever unless that's what works best for you. Even I don't stay in ketosis all the time. I don't freak out if I have to dip out of ketosis for my daughter's birthday cake or we go out and we have pancakes. I want to still live my life, I don't want to go live in a cave and only eat keto-friendly foods and never be tempted to eat processed carbs again—that's not fulfilling to me. I see the importance of a keto lifestyle, but at the same time I'm not dogmatic or religious about it. And I want you to know that there are different approaches to incorporating keto into your life depending on your goals. *You* get to choose! That's part of the adventure!

Maybe all this freedom to choose for yourself feels overwhelming rather than exciting. I know a lot of us don't feel like it's worth it to spend this much time on ourselves. The other day I spoke with a woman in her sixties who said something similar. She mentioned she had a couple of health concerns that were scaring her. When I asked if she'd seen her doctor she told me, "Honestly I don't think I'm worth the money or the effort. That money could be better spent." This idea that we must be selfless affects so many of us doesn't it? But you know what I saw very clearly in that moment? I saw her grandchildren playing near her and her daughter sitting in the other room. It was so clear to me right then and there how selfish it can be when we *don't* take care of ourselves! Her kids and grandkids want her around healthy and happy for as long as possible. *They* think she's worth it. Let me tell you in all caps: SELF-CARE IS NOT SELFISH. Taking care of your physical, mental, and spiritual health is not selfish.

I'll tell you what I told her: *you are worth it.* Yes, it may take some time to figure out what long-term approach to keto works for you. But it's worth it because you are worth it. I know that keto changes people's lives because I hear from people like Brooke, who found that "keto gave me something I could be good at. It gave me a way to feel really good about myself," and Chase, who said that keto helped him love his life again. My goal here is to help you feel as good for the rest of your life as you did on the 30-day program, because you deserve it. You are worthy of living a long, healthy life and you deserve nothing less!

TROUBLESHOOTING

If you've followed my plan closely for the full 30 days and you don't feel optimal, what does that mean? It might mean a couple of things. First, it's possible that you are in the small minority of people for whom the macros I used for my meal plans—75/20/5—don't work, and therefore you never got into a state of ketosis. Testing in the beginning should have helped clarify whether or not you were in ketosis, but if you didn't test for whatever reason, you may not know. Try the plan again and make sure to test. If you're still not in ketosis, you may want to find your fat, protein, and carb threshold using the methods I describe in "Testing for Ketosis Long-Term." Second, you may need to be on the keto cleanse phase for longer so that your body becomes fat-adapted—30 days works well for most people, but for some people it can take 60 or 90 days, so if you're not feeling great, try staying with the cleanse longer. If you've ruled out the other possibilities, and you still aren't feeling optimal, you may have an underlying condition that's surfacing now that you're eating clean, so I recommend you make an appointment to see your doctor.

EXTENDED FASTING

If you loved the fasting days in my program (Day 1 and Day 30), that's something you can incorporate into your life as well. I fast two to three times a year because I've found it to be the best cleanse I've ever done—better than other cleanses where you're running to the bathroom multiple times a day just to cleanse your body. Newsflash: your body can cleanse itself! That's what your liver and your kidneys are for. Fasting is a great way to help your body cleanse.

As an athlete growing up I was told that not eating is awful: it slows you down, you lose your muscle mass, your body will go into starvation mode and just store fat—I was told and believed all these myths about fasting. Plus, I used to have to fast once a month for 24 hours for religious purposes and I used to hate it. I would even stay up until midnight the night before eating as much as I could so that I wouldn't be as hungry the next day. Obviously, this wasn't the smartest approach and I didn't respect or understand the fasting process at that age. Now that I understand the physical, mental, and spiritual benefits of it, though, I love to do it. Well I shouldn't say I love to do it, let's be real . . . I love food. But I see the benefits of it and I do it for those reasons.

I do anywhere from a three-day up to a seven-day fast a couple times a year. It's a great way for me to not be a slave to food, to feel more in touch with my body, and to realize that we don't need food as much

as we think. Letting my mind control my body is huge—we let our bodies control us all the time but it's good to show our bodies who's boss.

Remember all those spiritual, mental, and physical benefits of fasting I discussed in Part 3? They are also relevant when it comes to long-term fasting: cell regeneration, better digestion, anti-aging properties, cleansing your body, the mental boost you get from knowing that you can go a day or two and still survive and feel optimal, and knowing you have the discipline and mental strength to control your body rather than having your body control you. We're taught to eat three square meals every day of our lives, and for me to know that I've been able to go seven days without food and still be a dad, an entrepreneur, and do all the things I need to do in a day is very empowering. It's fascinating to know that your body can survive without food.

I find the spiritual aspect very rewarding, too: becoming more in tune with your body can also get you more in tune with your spirit. Meditation is great on a fast, as is getting out in nature. You do feel connected to a higher power while fasting—I've even experienced euphoric feelings while fasting that have been very spiritually rewarding for me.

If you do decide to incorporate fasting into your life, remember to be safe about it. Make sure you stay hydrated and follow all the recs I detailed in the program.

REINTRODUCING DAIRY AND NUTS

I promised I wouldn't leave you without dairy and nuts forever! But I want to teach you how to reintroduce them safely and gently so that you stay feeling great. First, plan to take your time with it and do some self-experimenting. You've avoided these foods for 30 days and you don't want to shock your body with an ice cream binge or anything too wild. Keep in mind that you're trying to figure out the ideal diet for you, and so this reintroduction phase is all about gathering information.

Reintroduce dairy separately from nuts to allow your body a few days to see how it feels, and so that you can identify what, if anything, is giving you any reactions or symptoms. I recommended starting with dairy first. If, after the 30 days is up, you want to go back to dairy, use higher quality dairy if possible: milk and cheese from grass-fed cows, organic cage-free eggs, etc. Take two to three days of eating small amounts daily and reassess how you feel after consumption. Then do the same with nuts: re-implement nuts once a day and listen to how your body feels.

Adverse reactions might include bloating, gas, digestive issues, skin reactions, mood changes, lethargy, or major changes in sleep. If you do notice a reaction, most likely you have an intolerance to those foods. It DOES NOT mean you can never have those foods in your life—it just means that you are now empowered with this information and you get to decide how often you want to bring those foods back in. For me, for example, I know that I'm lactose intolerant, but that doesn't mean I never eat ice cream. It means I go into it knowing that this is going to suck for my digestion but at the same time it's going to taste good, so that's the choice I make every now and then. The most important thing is that you take it slow and listen to your body for two to three days consistently—you might be okay with both, and if so, feel free to continue having them. If not, then you decide where and when to bring those things back into your diet.

TARGETED KETO DIET

The Targeted Keto Diet has been around for some time and is popular with people who do CrossFit, jiujitsu, and other very glycolytic types of workouts. Hold on there, did you say "glycolytic"? I did. What I mean by *glycolytic* is workouts where you have to use full force, like a sprint or a burst of high energy from your body. Running a marathon is not a sprint, so it's not very glycolytic (not that it's not super challenging in other ways, though; much respect to all of you marathon runners!). When you're doing something all out for short periods of time, your body actually needs some glucose in those situations, and if you don't have enough, then you can feel a dip in performance. So that's why it's important to get keto-adapted first before you experiment with the Targeted Keto Diet,

TARGETED KETO DIET: A DAY IN THE LIFE

HERE'S AN EXAMPLE OF WHAT A DAY MIGHT LOOK LIKE ON THE TARGETED KETO DIET:

MEAL 1

FIRST:	PRE-WORKOUT:	POST-WORKOUT:
DREW'S PHAT COFFEE	½ CUP BLUEBERRIES	½ SWEET POTATO
	1 HARD-BOILED EGG	1 LOW-SUGAR BEEF STICK
	113 calories	157 calories
	5g fat, 11g carbs, 7g protein	2g fat, 20g carbs, 16g protein

MEAL 2

KETO COBB SALAD

INGREDIENTS:
GREENS: SPINACH, KALE, CHARD, BRUSSELS SPROUTS, AND BROCCOLI

PROTEIN:
1 HARD-BOILED EGG, GRASS-FED BEEF, AND SMOKED SALMON

FATS: GOAT CHEESE, GUACAMOLE, ALMONDS

LIQUIDS: HALF A LEMON, DASH OF APPLE CIDER VINEGAR

MEAL 3

RIB EYE STEAK	ASPARAGUS	EGGS

NUTRITIONAL INFORMATION FOR THE DAY

1,752 CALORIES,
129G FAT, 55G CARBS, 100G PROTEIN (40G NET CARBS)

so your body is efficient at using ketones and can switch back and forth between ketones and glucose well.

The protocol for Targeted Keto is to consume 5 to 15 grams of carbs about 30 to 60 minutes before a workout to fuel you, and the same amount of carbs 30 to 60 minutes post-workout to replenish those glycogen stores in your muscles and to help with recovery. The rest of the day you're sticking with the keto diet. So you're specifically timing your carbohydrates around your workouts to fuel yourself and then to replenish to help with things like muscle recovery from those types of exercises.

Some people like to use dextrose or maltodextrin powders for a quick and easy form of carbohydrate that's converted to energy really fast, and I'm okay with that, but personally I like to eat my carbs rather than drink them! So I eat small amounts of sweet potato or rice before a workout and after. The best kinds of carbs to add are fruit, sweet potato, potato, and rice—in other words, healthier forms of carbs. I mean, yeah, you could get your glucose from gummy bears, but why not go for the healthier, more satiating foods? Keep in mind that 5 to 15 grams of food is a small amount—approximately half a cup.

These carbs will give you that boost of energy—like rocket fuel on top of jet fuel—you need to be able to perform at those high intensity levels for short periods of time, but have no fear: your ability to switch over to ketones after burning that glucose is already at its peak from being fat-adapted.

If you want to give this approach a try, I recommend playing with it for about 30 days (after the 30-day cleanse) to see how your body reacts, especially if you do high-intensity interval training or sprints. You obviously might dip out of ketosis for a short period of time, which is totally fine because your body is really good at getting back in once it burns through that glucose. It won't suffer or struggle as much getting back into ketosis in these situations because you're already keto-adapted. Test your blood ketones to be sure that you're returning to a state of ketosis. You might notice that your ketone levels are low post-exercise, but that's normal as your body is using most of them to fuel you during a workout. No worries, though, as your body will continue to make more ketones (more fat burning . . . yay!!!) throughout the day.

This is your chance to become your own self-experimenter to find what works best for you. If you try this approach and don't like it, or if you read the above and say, NOPE, that does not sound like me, that's okay. There are other approaches to this lifestyle that I'll talk about next.

CYCLICAL KETO DIET

The Cyclical Keto Diet is more of a maintenance or balanced way to do keto. If you want to stay keto most of the time and you're not trying to lose fat anymore and you just want to maintain, I would stick with this approach, although you can still see some great results with fat loss on this approach as well if you stay disciplined with it and keep your calories within a reasonable range (1,400 to 1,600 for most women and 1,700 to 2,000 for most men). It's a great way to keep what you achieved in the detox phase but have more flexibility in your diet. This isn't the quickest way to lose fat on keto, but it's an awesome maintenance phase if you're happy with where you are but don't want to go back to a high-carb diet full-time.

You can still see some good gains with this approach if you want to put on some muscle mass without being strict 100 percent of the time. In order to gain muscle mass on the Cyclical Keto Diet, you need to be at a calorie surplus, more than 1,600 for most women and more than 2,000 for most men, and you need to be lifting heavy things. You also might want to experiment with higher levels of protein if your goal is to put on some lean muscle mass. Don't forget to test those blood ketones, though, to see if you're still in ketosis with this approach.

The basic protocol is that you have strict keto days and then you have "off" days where you get the majority of your calories from carbs instead of fats. I don't love the term "cheat day" because that suggests some guilt or being bad, but call your off days whatever works for you. Treat days, off days, refeed days, etc. There are as many different protocols as there are people! The most popular protocol for the Cyclical Keto Diet is five days on and two days off, or six days on and one day off. (Do I sound like Mr. Miyagi in *The Karate Kid*? Wax on, wax off. You get the idea.) It doesn't have to be five on and two off; it could be two weeks on and one day off whenever you want. You can even plan it out on your calendar and have a day to look forward to with your spouse, your kids, your friends. Maybe you have a picnic or party coming up or a vacation or anniversary and you want to have lots of carbs on those days. Whatever day(s) you choose, that's your day(s) to eat whatever you want to and—most important!—not feel guilt or shame about it. Look forward to those days. And don't feel bad the next day. You're fat-adapted, so your body already knows how to efficiently use ketones as a fuel source. That means that the next day you'll be right back on it with your *lifestyle* instead of "Oh, back on the DIET."

The one thing you want to avoid here is going high fat and high carb on your off days. Now, if you do it just one day a week it might not have too much of a negative impact, but doing high fat and high carb is actually bad for your body. A lot of the studies back in the day that demonized fat were based on high-fat, high-carb diets; they didn't factor in the high carbs that were in these meals, and that's why fat got a bad rap. But it wasn't actually the fat; it was the combination of fat and carbohydrates.

Imagine a teeter-totter or seesaw with carbs and fats on each end. Your protein stays the same, but when your carbs go up, your fats go down. Even though you're supposed to eat carbs on those days, you don't want to do high-fat foods like bacon on high-carb foods like pizza, or donuts dipped in chocolate. Small amounts of those are okay, but

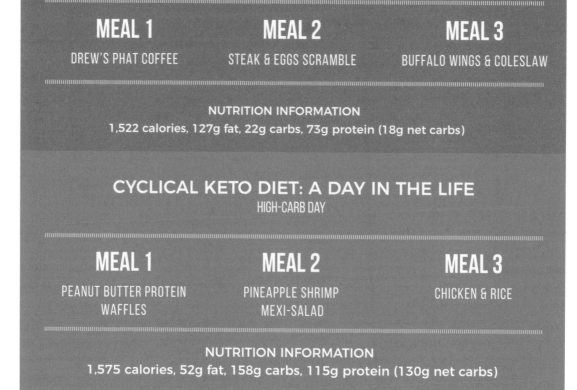

CYCLICAL KETO DIET: A DAY IN THE LIFE
HIGH-FAT DAY

MEAL 1

DREW'S PHAT COFFEE

MEAL 2

STEAK & EGGS SCRAMBLE

MEAL 3

BUFFALO WINGS & COLESLAW

NUTRITION INFORMATION
1,522 calories, 127g fat, 22g carbs, 73g protein (18g net carbs)

CYCLICAL KETO DIET: A DAY IN THE LIFE
HIGH-CARB DAY

MEAL 1

PEANUT BUTTER PROTEIN
WAFFLES

MEAL 2

PINEAPPLE SHRIMP
MEXI-SALAD

MEAL 3

CHICKEN & RICE

NUTRITION INFORMATION
1,575 calories, 52g fat, 158g carbs, 115g protein (130g net carbs)

don't go ham on these junk foods. I recommend healthier forms of carbohydrates that your body really likes, such as fruits, sweet potato, and rice. Because spoiler alert: there is not a lot of fat in those carbs either, plus they've got great micronutrients that will nourish your body!

If you want to continue the keto lifestyle, this is a good way to find balance with it and not have to feel guilty if you eat a carbohydrate—that is, you won't feel like it's the end of the world (I know from my pre-Fit2Fat2Fit days how dramatic we can be with our diets! Points at self.) You can find a healthy way to do this long-term, but make sure those carbs that you're eating are worth it. This isn't an excuse to have an epic cheat meal like the Rock would do—have you seen this on Instagram? Fifteen pancakes bigger than his head with butter and syrup and a side of brownies, or five pizzas with whiskey or tequila.

Look, you're not The Rock and neither am I. Hate to break it to you. He's been *super* strict for so long, and every once in a while he's like, I'm going to have one huge cheat meal. You don't need to be this way, unless you want to look like The Rock, which means you'll have to shave your head and get Polynesian tattoos (just kidding). Just realize that this isn't the last time you're going to have this food. You don't have to act like this is the last time you're going to have donuts or pastries or pancakes; there will be more opportunities to have these meals in the future, so don't feel that FOMO (fear of missing out), like I have to have all this food right now in massive quantities. You schedule those days so you know they'll come around again, so you don't have to eat every ice cream sundae that exists in the world, because they will be there waiting for you on the next round, I promise!

INTERMITTENT KETO DIET

This Intermittent Keto Diet protocol uses my keto program as a detox or cleanse phase. Maybe you notice carb or sugar cravings sneaking back up again and want to try and get rid of them with another 30-day detox; maybe you see really good results and don't want to live on keto but want to refresh those results a few times a year. This would also be a good protocol for people who tried for 30 days, saw some good results, but found it too challenging this time around, and instead of throwing this book out the window, you want to try again in a few months with a plan to be stricter or more disciplined with it! If this is you, I'm proud of you! (And thanks for not throwing my book.)

This approach works just as well for someone who has a healthy, balanced lifestyle already but who maybe every once in a while wants to do a keto cleanse or detox to lose that excess five pounds or so for a wedding or cruise, or for health reasons wants to make sure they're fueling their brain, heart, hormones, whatever, and they schedule a keto cleanse once or up to four times a year. It works well for people who do well on carbs. Maybe you are not insulin resistant and you can have a healthy lifestyle with carbs included, like some vegans and vegetarians. Does it work for everybody? No. Some people find that they just don't do well on carbs for whatever reason. Some people are the opposite—they don't do well on keto long-term! While everyone can benefit from getting their bodies into a state of ketosis, I know lots of people who don't thrive on a keto diet in the long term, and it's fine. Do my 30-day cleanse a couple of times a year to give your body a great reset, and then go back to your regular healthy diet if that's what works best for you. Bioindividuality is a beautiful thing. We don't have to think that my way is going to work for everyone just because it works for me. I don't know what's best for you—only you do.

This is a really fun approach to do with a community: friends, work buddies, or even family. Gather a group together to do Drew's 30-day Complete Keto challenge, and maybe even offer prizes for whoever loses the most weight or whatever your goal is.

TESTING FOR KETOSIS LONG-TERM

If you do choose to do keto, whether it's a cleanse a few times a year or staying strict keto most of the time, it's important to know that what worked for you yesterday might not work for you today or six months from now. Those macros of 70/25/5 don't need to stay that way forever. Your body will change over time, and your ability to get into and stay in ketosis will change. The way I do keto now is different from the way I did keto three or four years ago when I got started. It's going to be different for each person. For example, I've been doing it so long and I'm so fat-adapted—plus I work out every day (well, not every day, but maybe four to six times per week) and I have more muscle mass than your average person—that my ability to get into ketosis is a lot quicker, and so I have the ability to eat more carbs and more protein and still stay in a state of ketosis and feel fine. I can eat 50 to 75 grams of carbs on certain days and still stay in a state of ketosis.

So once you're fat-adapted, if you find you're losing strength in the gym or just not feeling as good as you were before, it's a good idea to find out what your carb threshold and protein threshold are, because they may have changed. Maybe in the beginning 70/25/5 worked for you but that may not work for you anymore, so it's time to change up your macros by upping your protein or your carbs, because that might be a more optimal state for you now that you've perhaps become stronger, lost more fat, gained more muscle, and increased your resting metabolic rate. You do that by testing your blood ketones with testing strips.

To find your protein and carbohydrate thresholds, you slowly increase your intake of them while testing your blood ketones along the way. Go one at a time. Let's say you start with your protein threshold. If you've been eating 80 grams strict protein per day for the last month or two months, slowly increase your protein day by day—from 80 to 85—and then test. If you're still in ketosis, go on to 90 and then test. And so on. Remember that anything above .5 mmol is nutritional ketosis. When you get to the point where you're test shows below .5 mmol and you're out of nutritional ketosis, you've found your protein threshold. Let's say you get to 90 or 100 grams of protein and then you get kicked out of ketosis, that's your protein threshold. Same thing with carbohydrates. Maybe in the beginning you started with 30 grams or less per day and you were strict, but now you've become so efficient at using ketones that you can change that number. Test the same way: increase from 30 to 35 and test, and so on. Maybe you find that between 40 and 50 is your sweet spot, so now you know you can get away with more carbs and more protein, lower your fat a little bit, and feel more optimal in the gym, have higher performance, increase your ability to build muscle mass and your ability to burn more fat as well, and you've got better energy but still stay in ketosis.

It's important to know what your protein and carbohydrate thresholds are; each person is going to be different, and your thresholds may change over time, so testing will empower you to make keto work for you. If you're doing keto long-term, I recommend testing every three to four months for about a week to see how your new approach is affecting ketone levels. Even if you're only doing the Intermittent Keto Diet, it's possible that the second time around doing keto your body will have changed and you don't need to be so strict.

HACKS FOR OVERCOMING EMOTIONAL CHALLENGES LONG-TERM

All the tips I mentioned for getting started on keto in Parts 1 and 2 will help you in your journey with keto long-term: the importance of having a support group, staying accountable, ditching the scale, not comparing yourself to others, not having tempting junk food in the house, meal prep and planning, meditation, practicing gratitude, and positive affirmations. Hopefully after the 30-day program you've incorporated a bunch of these hacks into your life and you're seeing the rewards of making keto an emotionally supported journey as much as one that's full of delicious food!

But the truth is that ending a detox and embarking on the rest of your life requires its own emotional support. You may be feeling overwhelmed at the idea of self-experimenting and becoming your own keto expert; or maybe you're feeling really excited to get back to the way your diet used to be before you started keto, only to find that you start feeling like crap after that first big plate of pasta or bowl of what used to be your favorite cereal, and now you don't know what the heck to do. Too often diet and health books give you a great 30-day plan, but then don't help you navigate what comes next at all. It's like my friend once complained to me about women's pregnancy books—there are tons of books about the three trimesters but almost nothing on, you know, being responsible for another human being for the rest of your life! A program is just that: a program. Now how do you make keto a *lifestyle*? By now you probably know I'm going to say that it's not just about the food. It's about your emotional and spiritual health as much as it's about your physical health. So here are my keto hacks for overcoming emotional challenges with food long-term:

1. Trust the process—and yourself!

When thinking about living keto long-term, don't think about *the rest of your life*— as in, for *the rest of my life* this means I'll never eat another donut—think about one day at a time. You already know so much more than you did 30 days ago! Trust that you'll continue to grow on the journey.

You'll become more familiar with foods in certain situations where right now you may feel like, what am I supposed to eat in this situation? You'll learn and grow, and sure, you may have some ups and downs, but in time you'll find what works for you. It's an exciting time! Soon you'll be on Pinterest looking up all the keto snacks and desserts for your kids and impressing everyone at the cookout with your amazing culinary skills. You know how to eat keto now, and you have all the tools you need to live keto, so trust the process and yourself!

2. Try intuitive eating

Intuitive eating. I'd heard this phrase for a few years before I actually understood it. I think it's because during my Fit2Fat2Fit days my intuition told me I wanted Cinnamon Toast Crunch, and so I thought I couldn't trust my intuition to steer me toward foods that were good for me. But I was wrong—it wasn't my intuition that wanted Cinnamon Toast Crunch, it was my body craving carbs and sugar! I was actually a slave to my food cravings when I constantly ate those foods. My intuition had nothing to do with it.

Now I understand that intuitive eating is all about developing a healthier relationship with food. Perhaps at the end of the 30-day program you're really feeling like you're missing some things—maybe your favorite brand of bagel with cream cheese or your favorite cake. So let's say you go ahead and have some. Rather than binging, try taking just one or two bites. I bet you'll realize, you know what? I don't need to eat this whole thing. I feel good with just one or two bites. Or maybe you'll even realize your joints, your gut, your brain don't feel that great when you eat those foods anymore, and then you say, well, not worth it. It is awesome and empowering to be able to have that control over your body! But we have to train our minds, too, so we can overcome that emotional eating mentality that says, "I need to eat all of this right now even if it makes me feel like crap!" If you practice listening carefully to your body, it will tell you when it doesn't like what you're feeding it, especially after 30 days of feeling fantastic.

It's important to note that I'm not saying you should beat yourself up if you eat cake or bagels. There should be no guilt and shame when it comes to eating food. You can't "mess up" or "fail" at intuitive eating. It's all just a process of learning to listen to your body and realizing that you're in control of your eating habits. You don't have to be a victim to your cravings. Food is more than just weight gain and weight loss. Food is *information* for your body. It affects us at the cellular level, it affects our hormones, our personality, our mood, how well we sleep, and so much more. That old saying you are what you eat? It's true. Food changes you at the core of who you are. So learn to get in touch with what makes you feel good and what makes you feel bad.

3. Stay mindful

Put all that meditation practice to good use in your long-term keto journey! Remember I said that meditation isn't about achieving bliss while meditating but about how it affects you in the rest of your life? Well, that goes for eating, too! Does this sound familiar: snacking on foods without even thinking about what they are because you're bored; eating while on your phone or watching television and not even tasting the food, it's just kind of there but not there; eating while at your desk working or popping something in your mouth as you drive? I bet that sounds like all of us at some point or another. That's called mindless eating.

It's important to be present in the moment with our food. When we're present as we eat, we can be in touch with what we're eating so we can listen to our bodies and practice intuitive eating. It helps us say, "Hey, this isn't really that good for me, I don't feel good," or "I'm really full, I should probably stop eating now." I know it is hard in the society we live in to eat mindfully. We're so pressed for time and we're so encouraged to be pressed for time. We have to be in a million places at a once and we just need quick energy. But it's time to slow down and be more present in the moment, and if we can do that we will have a better relationship with food.

4. Don't be a jerk!

When doing keto long-term you might quickly become that person who brings keto desserts or snacks to the party because you want to spread the word (or just because you want to have something you can eat!). People are naturally curious when they see someone eating in a way that's not the typical American diet. You may get all kinds of questions: "Oh, why are you eating so much fat?" or "Why are you putting butter in your coffee, that's weird!" or "I've heard about keto, my aunt did it," and so you suddenly become the voice for it. Congratulations, you're officially a representative of this way of eating! Badges and membership cards go out in the mail every six months (just kidding). Keto is a great conversation starter, but here's the thing: maybe *you* picked to stick with it for the rest of your life and that works great for you, but don't become preachy about it. Don't become dogmatic and look down on people, like, "Oh, carbs, that's so 1970s. Who eats carbs anymore? I haven't had them in twenty years, what's wrong with you?"

I know it's tempting to preach the good word of keto when you feel so amazing and you want others to feel great too, but the only thing that will come of that attitude is you will feel more isolated, and that won't support your keto journey. You want to feel part of a community, not a bossy person who no one wants to hang out with! If it works for you, that's great, people will gravitate to you. You don't need to tell people they should be doing this too. Instead, people will be like, "Wow, you look amazing! What are you doing?"

5. Find your happy balance— and know that it will change

What's *your* happy balance when it comes to diet, lifestyle, and physical health as well as mental and spiritual health?

Some people say they want to have the body of a Greek god, but in order to do that you're going to have to sacrifice *a lot* of personal time and other things that bring joy to your life. Do you know how strict you have to live to maintain that body? If we're being honest, for so many of us that's not the way we want to live. We want to go out and have drinks with our friends on Saturday night or be able to go to Disneyland and partake of the food that's there with our family on vacation and not feel like we can't live—and that's okay. Nothing wrong with that!

Whatever your happy balance is, that's okay, you just need to find out what yours is so that you realize the importance of maintaining a healthy body, mind, and spirit *and* being able to enjoy life. I see the world of biohacking, diet, and fitness going too far sometimes when the focus is that we have to do all these things, give up everything that makes life fun and enjoyable, just to squeak out a few more years of longevity or to look better in a bathing suit. Maybe that's what some people want, and if so, go for it! For me that doesn't leave enough room for life: cake at kids' birthday parties, trying something new while traveling abroad, sleeping in on Sundays. So find out what your happy balance is and let that include spiritual and mental health along with physical health. Let it include fun!

Then you need to be okay with it. Be at peace with whatever your happy balance is. Don't compare yours to anyone else's.

Know that you will need to reassess sometimes. If you have a baby or get surgery or your mother gets sick or you start a new job, or even if your body just changes and you need to change your macros or your workouts. Things change. So don't force your happy balance to be a static thing. Maybe think of your happy balance as a range, not a number, so you give yourself space for things to move. I know what my happy balance is when it comes to body fat, for example, but that happy balance sometimes goes through ebbs and flows, so my low is 10 percent body fat but my high is 14 to 15 percent because sometimes I'm stricter and sometimes I ease up. A range gives you some room to breathe.

6. Keep it interesting

Once or twice a year do something that you suck at. Seriously. It will help you take yourself less seriously! Pick something that challenges you and is outside your comfort zone, something you put money down on, like a Tough Mudder competition or a 5K or rock climbing class. This will challenge you to learn something new and forces you to train in a different way so you don't get stuck just doing three sets of 10 biceps curls every day for the rest of your life. There is no finish line. There is no destination. Come up with new, challenging ways to keep yourself engaged.

My first triathlon was a situation where I was kind of forced into it—a company that sponsors me wanted to fly me to Hawaii to do this triathlon. Now let me tell you: I'd never swum before. I mean, I went swimming for fun as a kid, but I never swam in a race before. I'd never done a bike race either. Nothing even close. I had two weeks to prepare. Two weeks!

I flew in the night before. I had my daughters with me. We got in at 10 P.M. Hawaii time, which is 2 A.M. Utah time, and we slept until 4:30 A.M. Hawaii time. I woke my girls, got them to the person who was going to watch them, and then pretty much was thrown to the wolves. Boom, they blew the whistle and I just ran into the ocean. I didn't die, but it was hard. Next up was the bike, and if you've never been on a bike for an extended period in a race before and suddenly you're on one for an hour and a half, that tiny little seat is up there really making you question your life choices.

When it was time to transition to running, my legs were like jelly. I wanted to be done. I wanted to stop and lie down on the ground. But I did it. I sucked at it but I finished—in 3 hours and 18 minutes. Not going to win any awards with that time, but you know what? I was glad I did it even though I sucked at it. I even signed up to do it the next year! Kind of like women who have a second baby even after they know what it's going to be like.

The second year I did a triathlon I trained really hard for it and I beat my time by only 13 minutes, which isn't bad, but it's not exactly major progress. I'm not going to be

a professional and I'm not going to win anything, but it's not about that. For me, it's rewarding to train for something that I suck at. That's what keeps people motivated long-term—even me, a fitness guy, gets burned out working out just to look good. If that's your why, it's not going to keep you interested very long. There's more to life than having a six-pack or having low body fat. So find a way to keep it exciting and interesting. I don't know if I'll ever do another triathlon; maybe next I'll take a Zumba class, surfing lessons, rock climbing—whatever it is for you, reinvent yourself to find a new passion as you evolve and learn and grow. Continually challenge yourself so you don't fall into your old ways, so you can be proud of yourself just for signing up and showing up. That means more than a number on a scale!

ROAD MAP FOR SUCCESS

We live in a results-driven, instant gratification society, there's no getting around that. I bet you originally picked up this book because that's what you wanted: RESULTS! Fair enough. From our grade school days of A students and F students to our trophy-obsessed sports culture and our weight-obsessed diet and fitness culture, we're all about celebrating results (and often shaming those on the losing end).

But I get to hear a different story when I talk with people who've done my programs. They lose weight, yes, but they also tell me how their perspectives shifted. What once was a weight loss program became something that helped them transform from being afraid all the time to feeling confident; I hear how they go from feeling worthless to full of self-love. I get to hear people talk about the "small" outcomes that really motivate them (aka non-scale victories): discovering a new love of eating healthy food or waking up invigorated rather than depressed. Or the outcomes they never expected, like getting their health back to the point where their doctor takes them off prescription drugs or leaving behind a lifetime of perpetual crash diets for a lifestyle that actually satiates and energizes them. This is complete transformation—complete keto!

I almost never get feedback about weight loss alone; what I hear time and time again is that my approach to keto changes lives, physically, emotionally, and spiritually. That what people find, myself included, is they no longer focus only on the goal of shedding pounds or getting shredded abs, but have learned to love the process—playing with their kids, discovering new recipes, becoming more efficient at work, clearer mind, not being a slave to food, sleeping better, going out and having fun with more energy and happiness. If we can flip the switch and focus on process over results, there is so much life we get to enjoy!

We won't completely transform if we're just chasing a number on a scale and/or a goal of fitting back into skinny jeans. That's all external validation, not change from within. If my Fit2Fat2Fit journey taught me nothing else, it's that weight loss and weight gain alone are not the full story. I thought I was on that path to learn how to lose weight, but what I really learned was how to truly listen when people shared their difficulties, not only with diet and exercise, but also with self-esteem and shame. I learned how difficult it can be to try losing weight when deep down you don't feel you deserve a better life and there's no one around to support you in the process.

And if my journey from falling apart to learning to love myself, not in spite of my vulnerability and weaknesses but because of them, taught me anything, it's that transformation cannot be about the body alone. There's a profound parallel between physical transformation and emotional and spiritual transformation. I believe that 100 percent. It's why I do what I do. As we transform ourselves emotionally and spiritually, the physical will follow. When we are focused only on physical transformation, there is no fulfillment. Sure, it's cool, but as Tony Robbins says, "Success without fulfillment is the ultimate failure." When we learn to love the process, by celebrating every healthy choice, every non-scale victory, every delicious meal, every newfound moment of energy and clarity, we own our story and we write our own happy endings.

My goal with this book you hold in your hands has always been to empower you to transform completely—that's why it's called *Compete Keto!* It's a diet program, of course, and it's a powerful one, with great nourishment, tons of tips and recipes, and good therapeutic gut, brain, hormone, and heart healing; but nothing is going to change unless you change your mind-set, you change your perception of food, yourself, health and fitness, and what your health and fitness look like.

For me, keto is so much more than a 30-day diet. It's a true lifestyle change—a physical, mental, emotional, and spiritual change. Yes, the keto diet is awesome: you'll feel physically amazing, and you'll experience all these awesome physical benefits. But I've found that what people struggle with is they think if they lose weight they'll be happy with themselves, or if they get fit they'll be happy with themselves, and this goes on and on forever: I'll be happy when [fill in the blank]. You have the power to change that mind-set. You can choose to be happy *now*; you can love yourself now while you're working on a better version of yourself. Why wait? Life is too short!

I've given you the physical tools to enjoy the journey with the keto diet, and the emotional and spiritual tools with positive affirmations and meditation, and this combination is what's going to help you achieve a higher level of happiness, self-love, and self-worth. This is your road map to success. Not just body, but mind and spirit also. Not just results, but learning to love yourself on the way. Over time you will have physical transformation, too, but the goal is not to have this amazing physical transformation yet be left empty inside, hating yourself, and not really achieving that self-love that you

deserve and that you're worthy of. The keto diet can be optimal for many people—your mental clarity, mental function, and gut health can all change for the positive with keto, not to mention it's delicious! It's highly therapeutic for your body on so many levels, in a way that's sustainable for a lot of people as a lifestyle change, and that is wonderful. But it's so much more than that. There's so much more to transformation than just weight loss. There are a million ways to lose weight; this isn't the only way to do it, and for you it may not even be the best way. I'm not here to preach that keto is the only one true way to lose weight, but it is a great way for many people. What I'm trying to say with Complete Keto and the keto lifestyle is that fitness and health are so much more than the physical transformation. The only way to know if this is the best way for you is to become your own self-experimenter and try it out for a minimum of 30 days to allow your body time to adjust.

If we can resist the message of our results-driven society and shift our perception to the journey itself, we'll realize the lessons are learned in the process. Get really interested in what you become during the process, like a little caterpillar on the journey toward becoming a butterfly. And the results? Let them fall where they may. The results will take care of themselves. You get to focus on the process of becoming a better version of you—and that is a beautiful opportunity. That is what Complete Keto is all about . . . becoming a Complete Human!

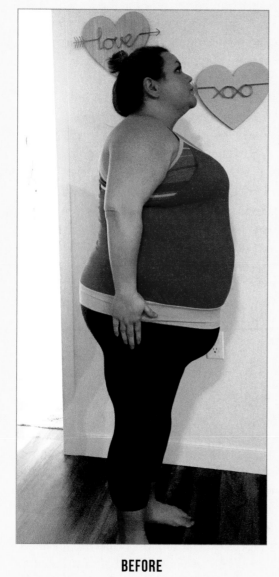

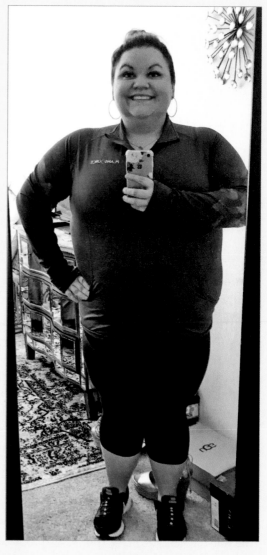

BEFORE

AFTER

KORTNI LISTER

I HAVE BEEN CHUBBY, FAT, PLUMP, WHATEVER YOU WANT TO CALL IT SINCE I WAS A KID. I remember being teased, but knowing that I couldn't do anything to change how my body looked.

Even with that, I never let my weight keep me from doing anything. I was a cheerleader in middle school, all-stars in softball, have run several 5Ks and 10Ks, trained for a half marathon (and injured myself lol), love hiking, pole fitness, TRX, etc. I love doing cartwheels with my nieces! I have a ridiculous amount of energy for a 35-year-old "obese" lady. Always have.

I have been dieting since I can remember. SlimFast, meal replacement bars, Weight Watchers, South Beach, Atkins, The Zone, Beach Body . . . etc. I was diagnosed with PCOS at 15. Then had a five-pound ovarian tumor extracted, along with an ovary and a fallopian tube at 16. When I was 24, I had LAP-BAND surgery as a means to an end. I lost about 40 pounds and my hair, skin, and nails looked rough. My organs were not fatty and I am not an overeater. This was quick to return once I could eat a non-liquid diet.

I was at a loss. My sister and I met a doctor who finally figured out that along with PCOS, we both have a reverse T3 and T4 hypothyroidism. Basically, we hit the genetics jackpot of how to hold on to fat for dear life. This amazing doctor put us on thyroid meds and modified HCG, to help jump-start the weight loss. I lost 34 pounds in three weeks . . . and became extremely ill. I was in immense pain, enough pain that I landed in the ER with what was diagnosed as a ruptured ovarian cyst. After 8 weeks, 4 ER visits, 6 doctors, countless tests, and $150,000+ in medical bills, I had lost 76 pounds and became septic. A wonderful surgeon decided to remove my gallbladder in an emergency surgery.

After all of this, the weight packed right back on and then some.

Fast-forward to four years later, and I have never felt better. My sister DVR'd an episode of Dr. Oz, where Drew Manning was talking about the Ketogenic Diet. At first, I thought, "Could this be real?!" Then after researching how Keto works, we made a plan to try it. Keto is THE ONLY thing to have ever remotely worked for me. Even without my gallbladder, Keto is the only way of life. It is not a diet; it is a lifestyle. I don't even have to think about it! It has become second nature . . . 75 percent fat/20 percent protein/5 percent carbs. Something so simple has changed everything. My acanthosis nigricans have almost disappeared, PCOS is under control, my thyroid is working. When I started Keto on January 2, 2018, I was wearing size 22/24 plus-sized clothing. As of today, June 8, 2018, I am wearing size 14/16 misses-sized clothing. I never thought this could be possible! 2018 is the year I get to take my life back from what became a life sentence at 15. I make new goals and challenges every day and am excited to make progress!

— KORTNI LISTER

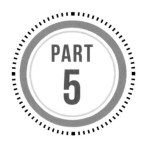

PART
5

EXERCISES

Reminder that when it comes to working out and exercise, in my opinion, it's NOT the most important component of getting in shape. Sleep, nutrition, and managing stress are way more important. You'll still see great results following the CK30 program and just going for a walk and being active every day. With that said, if you want to maximize their results and already enjoy working out, then you'll love the CK30 workouts! In the pages ahead, I'll explain and illustrate how to do each of the exercises in the program, including ways to modify each move in a way that works for your body.

When it comes to progress, sometimes we place SO much value on our scale weight, hoping to see that number go down week after week, but in reality there's so much more to becoming healthier than seeing that number go down on the scale. That's why I like to set people up for wins outside of just the scale. So, I designed the workouts to show your progress week to week even though you might not always see your efforts reflected on the scale. This workout program is designed to show you that you're getting stronger and faster week after week. Have fun!

AIR SQUATS

1. Stand with your legs slightly wider than shoulder width apart and toes slightly pointed out.

2. Sit back and down as if you were going to sit in a chair.

3. Lower down until your thighs are parallel to the floor, keeping your knees over your ankles.

4. Push back up through your heels to the starting position.

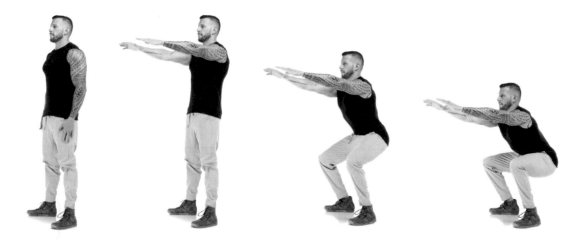

TIP: Feel free to put your arms directly out in front of you to help you balance your weight. Keep your chest up and don't round your back.

MODIFIED AIR SQUATS

Stand with your feet slightly wider than shoulder width apart, toes slightly pointed out, with a chair, bench, or couch behind you. Keeping your weight in your heels and your arms reaching out from your chest, lower down into a squat. Tap your butt onto the chair (or sit completely) and stand back up. As you stand back up, push your feet into the floor and avoid using your hands to press against your legs or chair to assist you. Do your best to use only your legs. If it's so hard you're falling onto the chair, get a higher chair.

To further modify, grab a partner and hold your partner's hands for support when sitting down and standing back up.

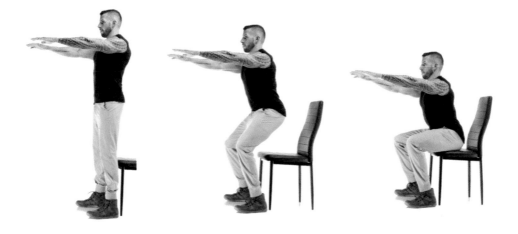

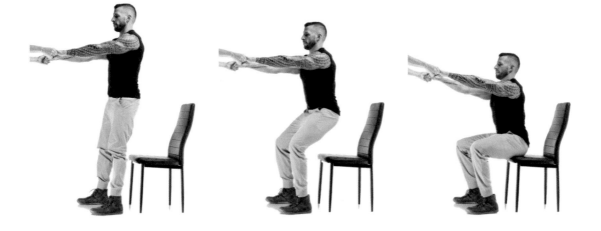

BURPEES

1. Stand with your feet hip width apart.

2. Lower into a squat position with your hands flat on the floor in front of you.

3. Kick your legs backward into a push-up position and lower yourself to the floor.

4. Push yourself back up and thrust both feet forward so you are back in the squat position.

5. Jump up and raise both hands over your head.

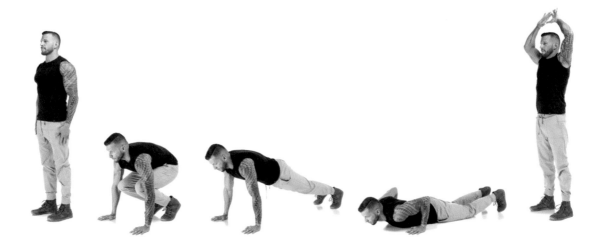

MODIFIED BURPEES

Get into a push-up position with your hands propped up on a chair, couch, or desk so your body is at a 45-degree angle to the ground. Jump or step both feet in toward your chest and then back out, repeating that process over and over again.

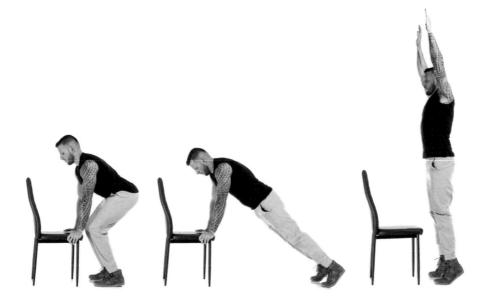

To further modify, do this same movement against a wall.

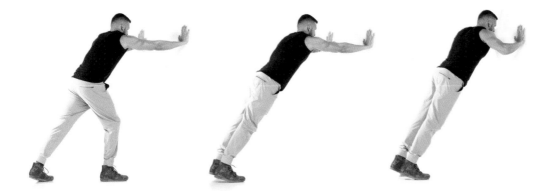

DIPS

Using a chair, bench, or step:

1. Place your hands shoulder width apart with fingers facing forward, elbows facing back, and feet extended in front of you.

2. Keeping your shoulders back, lower your body straight down 2–3 inches.

3. Raise your body back to starting position.

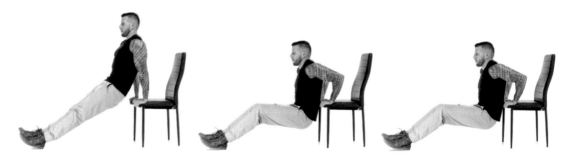

MODIFIED DIPS

Sit on the floor with your legs bent and feet flat on the floor. Place your hands back behind you with your fingertips facing forward. Bend elbows to a 90-degree angle in dipping motion, or as low as you can bend, then push back up, using your triceps muscles. Keep your elbows pointed toward the wall behind you.

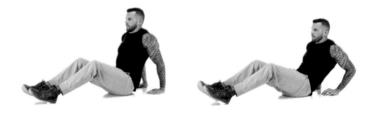

JUMPING SQUATS

1. Stand with your legs slightly wider than shoulder width apart and toes slightly pointed out.

2. Sit back and down as if you were to sit into a chair. Lower down until your thighs are parallel to the floor while keeping your knees over your ankles.

3. In the low position, quickly swing your arms down and slightly behind you, then swing them up as you explode into a jump. Land softly and right back into the squat position. Repeat.

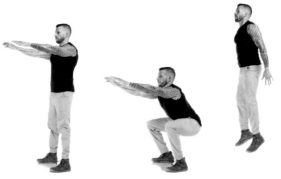

TIP: Your body should be straight up in mid air. Landing on your heels is bad for your knees. Landing on your toes protects the joints.

MODIFIED JUMPING SQUATS

Replace this movement with modified air squats, but feel free to add a toe raise at the end of it.

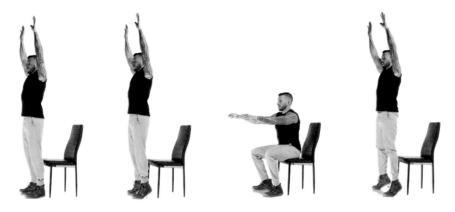

LEG RAISES

1. Lie down on your back on the floor.

2. With your arms at your sides, palms down on the floor, lift your feet slightly off the floor.

3. Keeping your legs straight, bring your legs up to 90 degrees, perpendicular to the floor, then lower back down until they hover just above the floor before bringing back up. You can tap the floor if necessary.

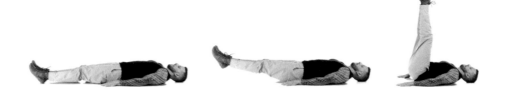

MODIFIED LEG RAISES

Lie down with your back on the floor, knees bent and feet flat on the floor. Place your arms next to your torso with palms flat on the ground. Lift your feet off the floor, engaging your abs. While keeping your knees together, bring your legs as close to your chest as possible, and then slowly bring feet back down to the ground.

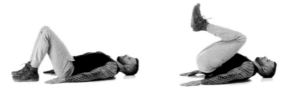

To further modify, sit in a chair and have your feet flat on the ground. Straighten one leg out in front of you and lift leg as far as you can off the ground, then slowly tap your heel on the ground. Repeat motion on opposite leg.

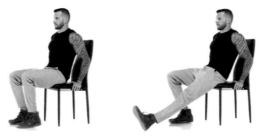

LUNGES

1. Step forward with one leg.

2. Lower down until both knees are bent at a 90-degree angle.

3. Push back to the starting position by pushing through your front heel.

4. Repeat movement with the opposite leg forward.

TIP: Keep your upper body straight, shoulders back, and core engaged. Keep your front knee directly above your ankle.

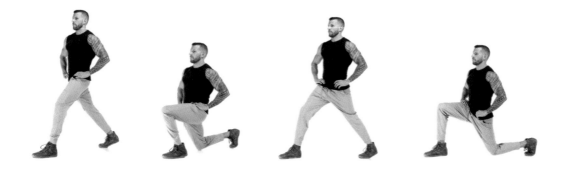

MODIFIED LUNGES

Using a chair or wall for stability, place one hand on the chair or wall and the other on your hip. Then step one leg forward and lunge down, bringing your back knee as far down as you feel comfortable. Be careful to not let your front knee go past your toes. Keep your chest upright. Then push off that front foot back to your starting position.

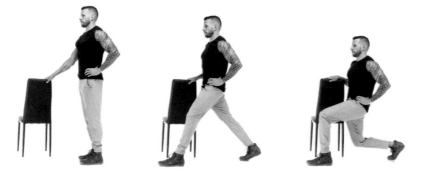

MOUNTAIN CLIMBERS

1. Start in a plank position.
2. Without rounding your back, pull one knee up and in toward your chest.
3. Straighten your leg back to the starting position.
4. Repeat movement with the opposite leg.

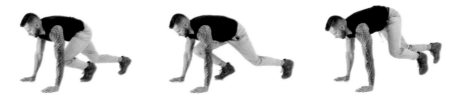

MODIFIED MOUNTAIN CLIMBERS

Get in push-up position with hands elevated on a chair, couch, or desk. Start with one foot forward, one foot back. While keeping your core tight and body in a straight line, perform a small hop and switch your feet in midair, bringing your front foot to the back and back foot to the front. Repeat.

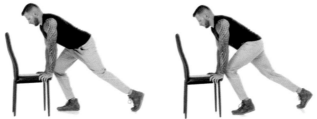

To further modify, start with both feet forward. Step one foot back and tap your foot on the ground with your leg fully extended, then bring it back forward. Switch legs and repeat. Continue alternating. Make sure and keep your core tight the entire time. Your body should be at a 45-degree angle the entire time.

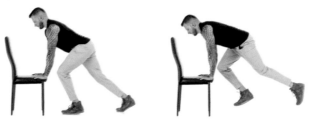

PUSH-UPS

1. Get into a standard push-up position, hands slightly wider than shoulder width apart.

2. Keeping your body in a straight line (squeeze your glutes and keep your lower abs pulled in to achieve this), lower down until your chest almost touches the floor, elbows pointed back at about 45 degrees from your body.

3. Push through your chest to return to starting position.

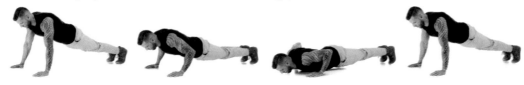

MODIFIED PUSH-UPS

Get in push-up position on the ground with hands about shoulder width apart. Drop to your knees so that just your knees and hands are touching the floor. As you keep your body in a straight line, bring your chest down as close to the floor as you can and push yourself back up to the starting position. Make sure your butt is not sticking up high in the air, and make sure your butt is not sinking low below your hips either. Squeeze your glutes and pull your abs in the entire time to keep this position.

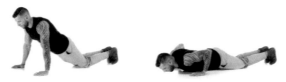

To further modify, place hands shoulder width apart against a wall. Step your feet back to about a 45-degree angle, or as far out as is comfortable to you. While keeping your body in a straight line by squeezing your butt and keeping your abs pulled in, bend your arms to bring your face as close to the wall as possible, then push back out again.

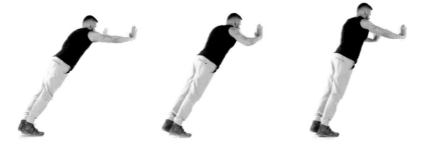

PLANK

1. Lie face down on the floor and prop yourself up on your elbows, keeping your elbows directly under your shoulders and your hips off the floor, and squeezing your glutes to keep your body in a straight line.

2. Create tension by using the resistance of the floor to "pull" your elbows and toes toward each other.

3. Breathe.

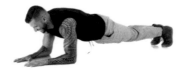

TIP: Remember to keep abs pulled in and glutes active to maintain a neutral spine.

SIDE PLANK

1. Lie on your side.

2. Create a straight line from head to feet, resting on your forearm. Your elbow should be directly under your shoulder.

3. With your abs gently contracted, lift your hips off the floor, maintaining the line.

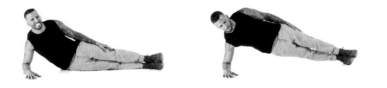

MODIFIED SIDE PLANK

Lie on your side with your elbow bent in a 90-degree position tucked under your shoulder and your forearm flat on the ground, perpendicular to your body. Lift your hips off the ground, squeezing your glutes and drawing your abs in, with your bottom leg bent in a 90-degree position. The top leg can be straight or bent. Your forearm and knee should be supporting your body weight. Make sure you breathe!

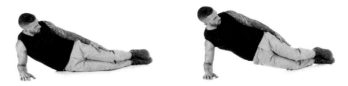

To further modify, stand perpendicular to a wall. Place one hand on the wall and walk your feet out until your body is at a 45-degree angle from the wall. You should feel your obliques and core engage to keep you at that angle.

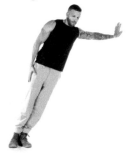

SIT-UPS

1. Lie on your back with your legs extended and your arms overhead.

2. While you keep your legs flat on the ground, engage your core and swing your arms forward to sit up until you reach a 90-degree angle.

3. Lower yourself back down to the starting position.

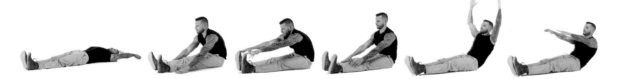

MODIFIED SIT-UPS

Lie on your back on the floor with your knees bent, feet flat on the floor. Keep your tailbone flat against the ground. Extend your hands up toward the ceiling and lift your upper body, squeezing your abs, lifting as high as you can before coming back to the starting position.

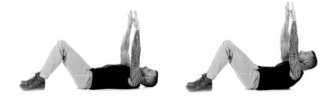

STEP-UPS

1. Stand in front of a bench, chair, or sturdy low table.

2. Step up, pushing through your heel and keeping your knee outside of your big toe.

3. Tap your other foot on top of the bench and bring it straight back down.

4. Bring the leg you stepped up with back to starting position; switch to step up with other leg and continue alternating.

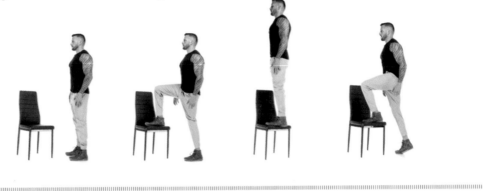

MODIFIED STEP-UPS

Place a small step stool against a wall or use a chair for support. Place one hand on the wall or chair for stability and step up onto the stool one foot at a time, then step down. The higher the step, the harder it will be. The lower it is, the easier it will be.

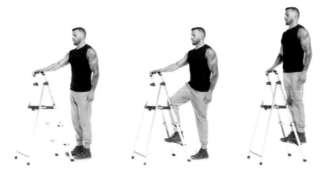

To further modify, place both hands on the wall for stability and step up, one foot at a time, then step down. You may also do this on a stair in your house or a curb.

SUPERMAN

1. Lie flat on your stomach with arms fully extended out in front of you (like Superman).

2. Lift both your legs and your arms slightly off the ground (about 6 inches).

3. While you hold this position, engage your glutes and lower back.

4. Release back down to the ground.

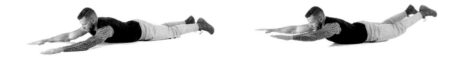

MODIFIED SUPERMAN

Lie on your stomach flat on the floor. Keep your legs out straight behind you, and your arms reaching forward. Lift your right arm and left leg as high as you can off the floor while your other arm and leg stay on the floor. Then switch and do the same with your left arm and right leg.

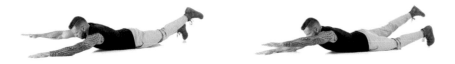

WALL SIT

1. Stand with your back resting on a wall behind you.

2. Lower down into a squat, thighs parallel to the floor or deeper, knees outside of big toes, pushing through your feet and into the wall behind you.

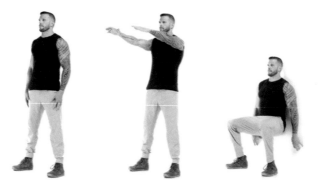

MODIFIED WALL SIT

Lean your back flat against a wall, and squat down as far as you can go. Make sure your feet are shoulder width apart, toes slightly pointed out. This can be modified to any level; determine which depth is best for you and hold that position.

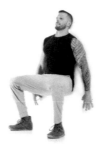

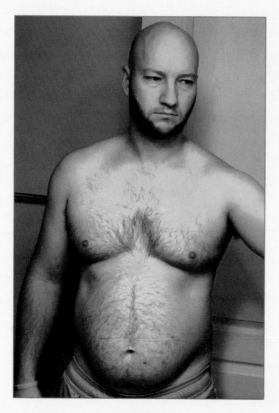

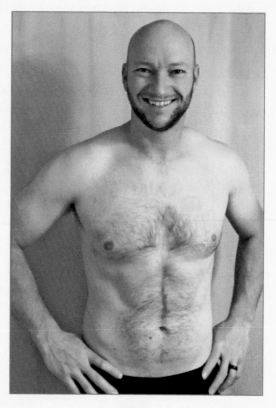

BEFORE

AFTER

JUSTIN FUCHS

MY FATHER PASSED AWAY IN HIS EARLY 60S WHEN HE HAD A STROKE CAUSED BY high blood pressure. He had very high blood pressure for as long as I can remember, and he did almost nothing to fix it and ate anything and everything that was sweet. Shortly before he passed I was getting a physical at the doctor's office when they told me I was 40 pounds overweight and had high blood pressure. After my father passed away, I knew I was on the same road that led him to an early grave, and I decided I had to make some lifestyle changes. I started working out, and got some results, but nothing close to the results I wanted. I tried a few different diets, counting calories, but I just felt hungry all the time and it wasn't something I could keep up indefinitely.

After a while I got discouraged and stopped dieting and working out. As a result, my blood pressure started to creep back up. I knew I needed something I could do for the rest of my life, so I could be healthy and be there for my kids and future grandkids when they are grown. I was talking with my older brother about it and he mentioned the Keto diet to me. I started doing some research and that's when I found Drew.

When I started January 1, I asked myself, is this really worth it? After three months on the Keto diet, I have answered that question many times . . . YES!!! I have lost a total of 36 pounds. I went from a size 36 pants to a size 30. I have more energy to play with my kids instead of just sitting on the sidelines and watching them play. I don't lose my breath and can run and keep up with them. But the best part is when I went back to the doctor's office and he took my blood pressure and asked who I was trying to impress because my blood pressure was so good!

The Keto diet has completely changed my life (and not just because I had to buy all new clothes). It has given me the promise of a better future with my family, one where I don't just sit on the sidelines watching because I don't have the energy, or I'm embarrassed to because of my weight. It is difficult and takes hard work and dedication, but it is 100 percent worth it!

— JUSTIN FUCHS

RECIPES

Here are all the recipes you'll find in the meal plan in Part 3, as well as every other recipe I've mentioned throughout the book. They are categorized by meal—breakfast, lunch, and dinner—and organized alphabetically so that you can find things easily.

There's also a section at the beginning on keto basics, with key foods like paleo mayo and keto hot chocolate, and a section with Cyclical Keto Diet recipes at the end. You can mix and match the lunches and dinners; I just wouldn't move breakfast around, because who really wants to have coffee for dinner and then be up all night from the caffeine? But if, for example, I've listed Day 1 as burgers and avocado and Day 2 as salmon, and it works better for you to have salmon on Day 1, that's fine.

If you do mix and match, realize that your macros for the day might not be what you see in the program portion of the book. They still should be similar, but not exact, so if you

mix and match just be sure to keep an eye on your macros for the day. Every recipe includes nutritional information that will enable you to do so. Please note that vegan and vegetarian recipes include net carb content (as well as total carbs) because on veg*n keto you'll be counting net carbs instead of total carbs.

I put these recipes together with a lot of love for simple, whole-food ingredients, the pleasure of connecting with loved ones over the dinner table, and the joy of eating delicious, satiating food. Whether you're new to cooking or you're a wizard in the kitchen, you are welcome at the keto table—I hope you have a blast trying new things and experimenting with keto cooking!

KETO

BASICS

KETO FLU KILLER
(DREW'S HOMEMADE ELECTROLYTE DRINK)

4 calories | 1g carbs

½ cup lemon juice

¼ teaspoon pink salt

½ teaspoon potassium citrate

2 tablespoons magnesium powder (magnesium citrate or glycinate)

¼ cup erythritol (or ⅛ cup stevia or monk fruit sweetener)

Combine all the ingredients in a large pitcher with 5 cups water and mix well. Start with drinking ½ to 1 cup per day. Do not chug; drink slowly.

KETO HOT CHOCOLATE

MAKES 1 SERVING

311 calories | 31g fat | 2g protein | 7g carbs (5g net carbs)

8 ounces unsweetened almond milk

2 tablespoons heavy cream

1 tablespoon butter

1 scoop vanilla MCT oil powder, such as Complete Wellness Vanilla MCT Powder

½ tablespoon unsweetened cocoa powder

Stevia or xylitol, to taste

Dash of cinnamon

Combine all the ingredients in a saucepan and heat until warm and mixed well. Once warm, place the hot chocolate into a blender and mix until frothy. Enjoy immediately!

PALEO MAYO

128 calories | 14g fat | 0g carbs | 0g protein

1 cup avocado oil

1 egg

1 teaspoon lemon juice

½ teaspoon Dijon mustard

¼ teaspoon sea salt

Combine all the ingredients in a mason jar.

Insert an immersion blender all the way to the bottom of the jar and turn it on high. Leave the immersion blender on the bottom of the jar for 30 seconds, until the whole bottom is white. Lift the immersion blender up to continue emulsifying. Continue blending until the mixture has thickened, about 1½ minutes.

Keep covered in refrigerator for up to 4 weeks.

PALEO RANCH DRESSING

MAKES 16 SERVINGS

134 calories | 15g fat | 0g carbs | 0g protein

1 cup paleo mayonnaise

¼ cup coconut milk, from a can

1 teaspoon apple cider vinegar

½ teaspoon onion powder

½ teaspoon garlic powder

1 teaspoon dried dill

1 teaspoon dried parsley

Sea salt and pepper, to taste

Mix all the ingredients together in a bowl until well combined. Keep in an airtight container for up to 1 week in the refrigerator.

SALT SHOT

½ teaspoon sea salt or pink salt

Sprinkle salt into the palm of your hand and dump it into your mouth. Then chug as much water as you can to wash the salt down.

KETO
BREAKFAST

DREW'S PHAT COFFEE

MAKES 1 SERVING

229 calories | 23g fat | 6g carbs | 0g protein

12 ounces coffee, brewed and hot

1 tablespoon ghee or coconut oil

2 scoops vanilla MCT oil powder, such as Complete Wellness Vanilla MCT Powder

Dash of cinnamon

Pinch of sea salt

Combine all the ingredients in a blender.

Mix until frothy.

Enjoy immediately!

NOTE:

Phat coffee does not work well iced; it will cause the coconut oil to solidify.

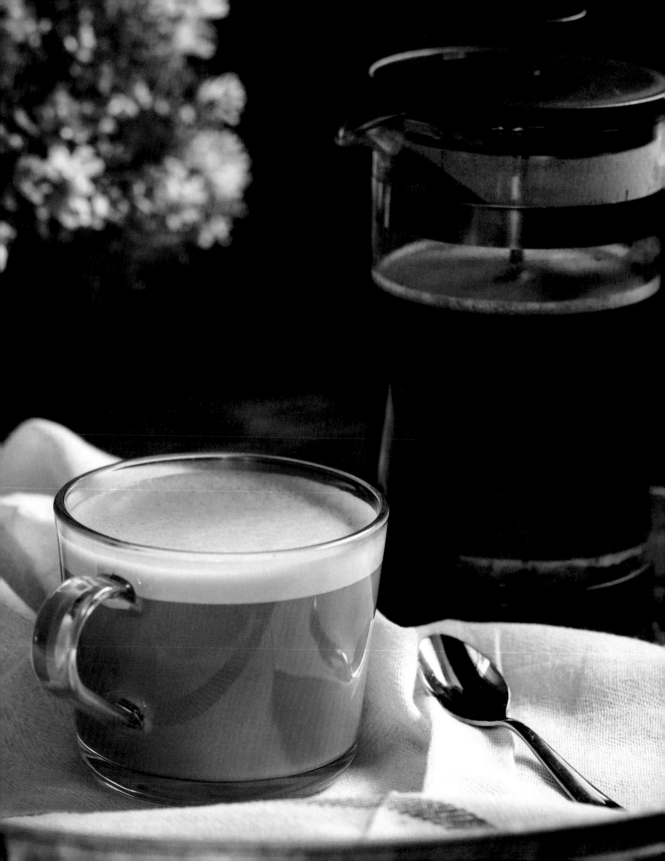

KETO
LUNCH

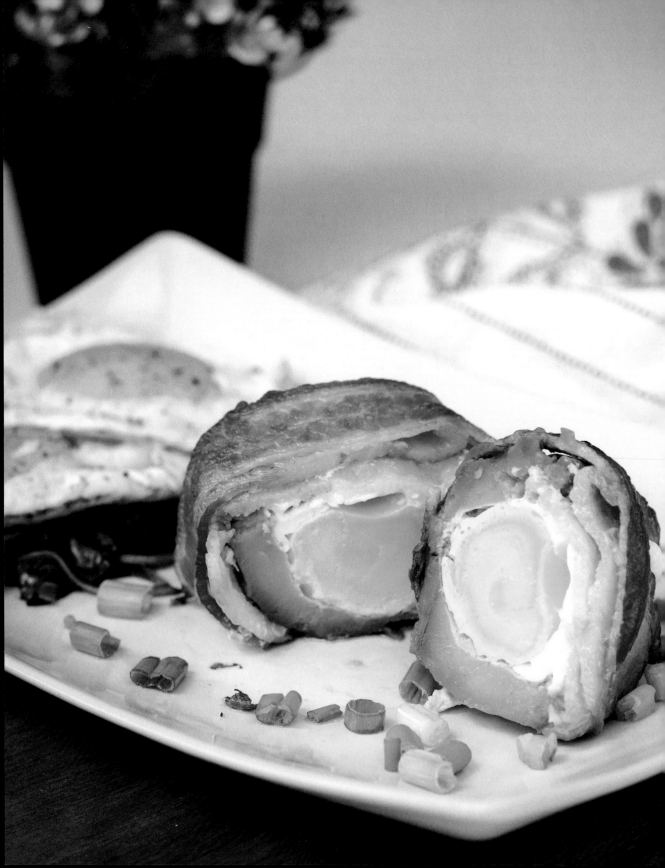

AVOCADO EGG BOAT

556 calories | 47g fat | 8g carbs | 27g protein

½ medium avocado

3 eggs

Sea salt and pepper, to taste

2 slices bacon

1 tablespoon ghee

1 cup spinach

Preheat the oven to 425 degrees.

Cut the avocado in half; remove the pit and skin, being careful to leave the fruit intact. Scoop some of the fruit out of the center so you have enough room for the egg.

Place the avocado in a muffin tin, with the center facing up. Crack the egg into the center and sprinkle with salt and pepper.

Carefully lift the avocado and wrap it with both slices of bacon.

Bake for 15 to 18 minutes, or until the egg is cooked and the bacon is crispy.

Meanwhile, melt ½ tablespoon of ghee in a pan, fry remaining eggs to desired doneness, and set aside.

In the same pan, melt the remaining ghee and sauté the spinach until it's just wilted, about 2 minutes. Place it on the plate.

Place the fried eggs over the spinach and serve with a bacon-wrapped avocado boat on the side. Enjoy!

BACON AVOCADO EGG SALAD WRAPS

MAKES 1 SERVING

641 calories | 58g fat | 8g carbs | 30g protein

3 hard-boiled eggs, chopped

¼ medium avocado, mashed

2 tablespoons avocado oil mayo

Sea salt and pepper, to taste

2 romaine lettuce leaves

4 slices of bacon, cooked and chopped

Combine the eggs, avocado, mayo, salt, and pepper in a small bowl. Mix until thoroughly combined.

Divide the mixture between the lettuce leaves, sprinkle with bacon, and enjoy immediately!

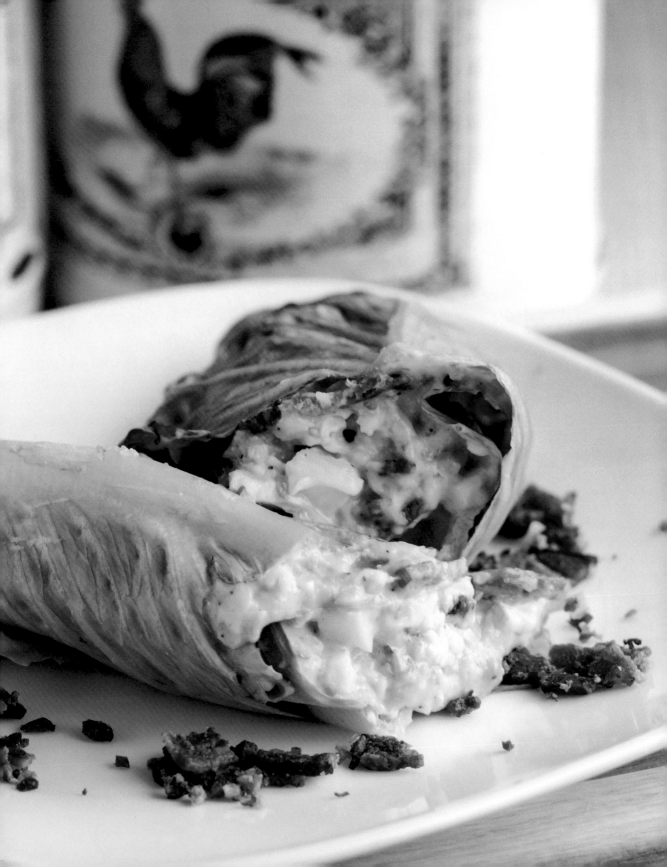

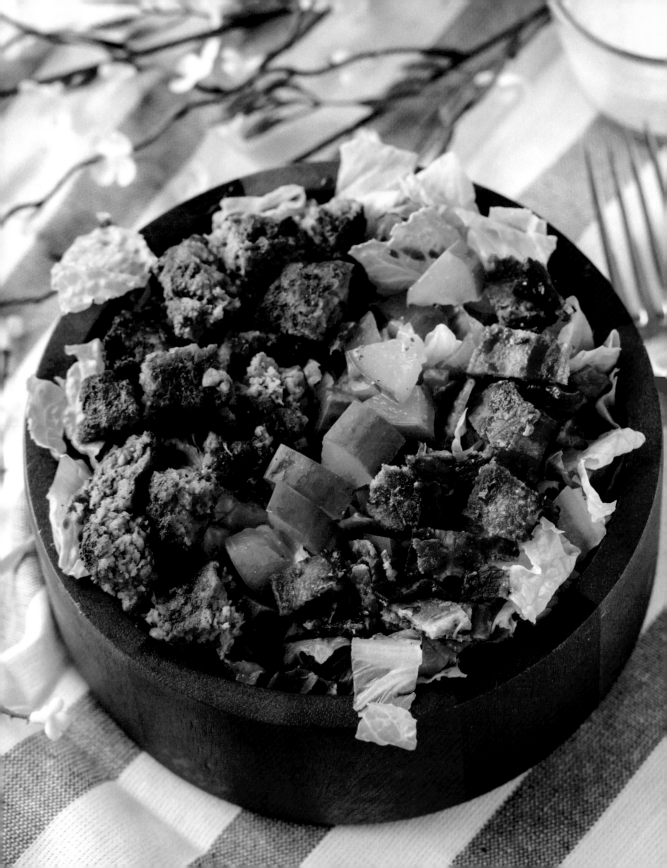

BACON BURGER SALAD

MAKES 1 SERVING

685 calories | 53g fat | 6g carbs | 44g protein

2 cups romaine salad mix, chopped

⅓ cup chopped pickles

5-ounce ground sirloin hamburger patty, cooked and cut in bite-size pieces

3 slices of bacon, cooked and chopped

FOR DRESSING:

2 tablespoons paleo mayonnaise

1 to 2 tablespoons white vinegar, to taste

1 teaspoon mustard

½ tablespoon pickle relish (no added sugar)

Dash of paprika

Pinch of stevia, to taste

Layer the chopped romaine, pickles, cooked hamburger patty, and cooked bacon in a large bowl.

Mix all the ingredients for the dressing in a small bowl.

Drizzle the dressing over salad and enjoy immediately!

BACON VEGGIE OMELET

MAKES 1 SERVING

595 calories | 47g fat | 7g carbs | 35g protein

1 tablespoon ghee

4 eggs

Sea salt and pepper, to taste

¼ cup chopped broccoli

1 cup spinach

¼ cup chopped onion

3 slices of bacon, cooked and crumbled

1 tablespoon guacamole

Melt the ghee over medium heat in a medium skillet and swirl the pan so the ghee coats the entire bottom of the pan.

In a bowl, beat the eggs together and season with sea salt and pepper.

Add the eggs to the pan and wait about 30 seconds to 1 minute until the edges begin to set. Then add the broccoli, spinach, onions, and bacon, sprinkling evenly over the eggs.

Once the eggs begin to bubble and become firm, after about 2 to 3 minutes, use a spatula to separate the egg from the side of the pan, and flip one side of the omelet over, folding the omelet in half.

Place the omelet on a plate, top with guacamole, and enjoy!

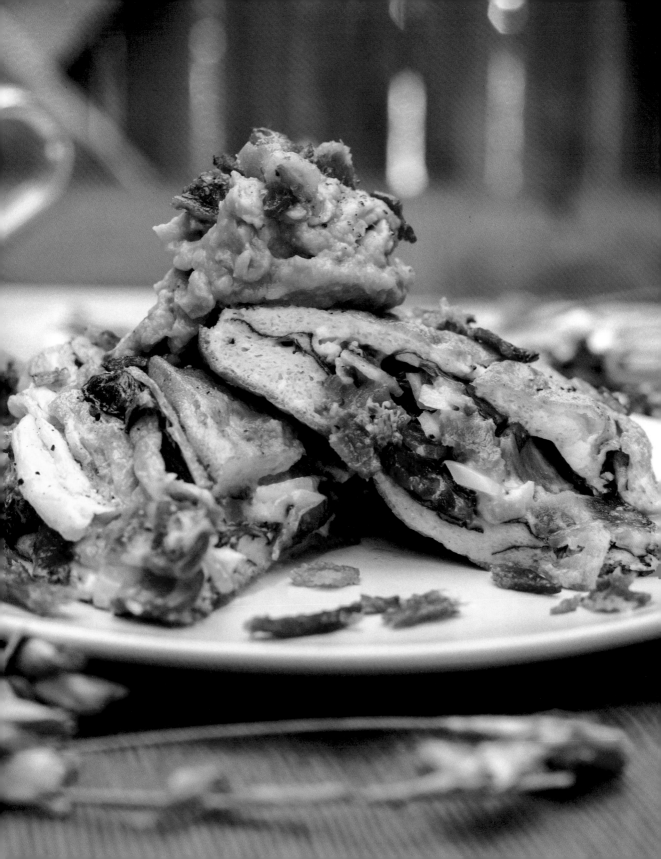

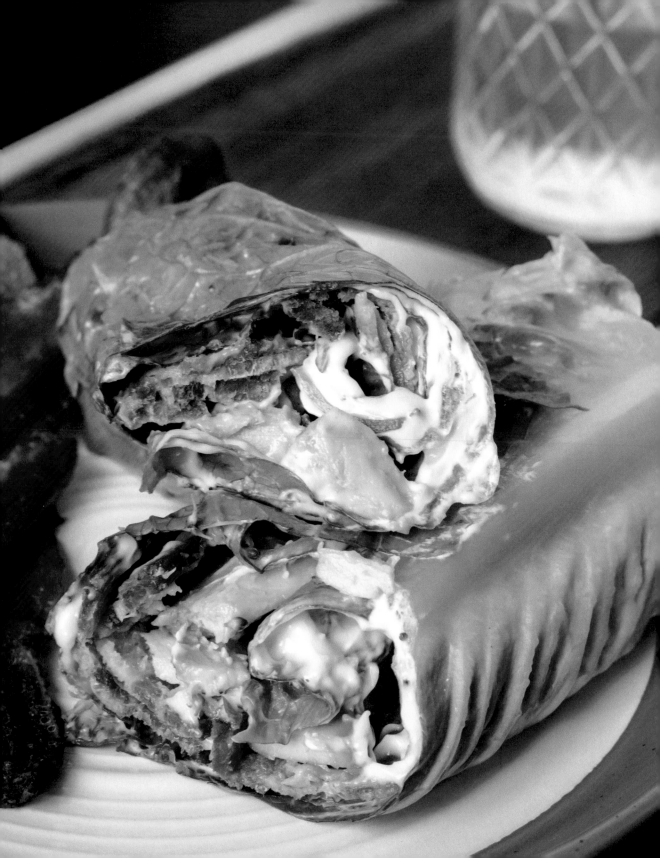

BLA (BACON LETTUCE AVOCADO) WRAPS

641 calories | 63g fat | 11g carbs | 22g protein

2 romaine lettuce leaves

2 tablespoons paleo mayo

8 slices bacon, cooked

½ medium avocado, sliced

Sea salt, to taste

Lay the lettuce leaves on a plate, and spread the mayo on each piece.

Divide the bacon between the lettuce leaves and top with the avocado.

Sprinkle the avocado with sea salt and enjoy immediately!

CAESAR CHICKEN SALAD

MAKES 1 SERVING

677 calories | 55g fat | 6g carbs | 36g protein

1 tablespoon avocado oil

3 ounces boneless, skinless chicken thighs

Sea salt and pepper, to taste

¼ teaspoon garlic powder

¼ teaspoon Italian seasoning

3 cups spring greens salad mix

⅓ cup chopped tomatoes

3 slices of bacon, cooked and crumbled

3 tablespoons hemp hearts

2 tablespoons paleo Caesar dressing

Drizzle avocado oil in a skillet over medium heat and add the chicken thighs. Toss until well coated. Season with sea salt, pepper, garlic powder, and Italian seasoning. Cook for 8 to 10 minutes until chicken is cooked through or reaches an internal temperature of 165 degrees Fahrenheit.

Layer the salad mix, tomatoes, chicken thighs, and bacon in a large bowl, and sprinkle with hemp hearts.

Drizzle Caesar dressing over the salad and enjoy!

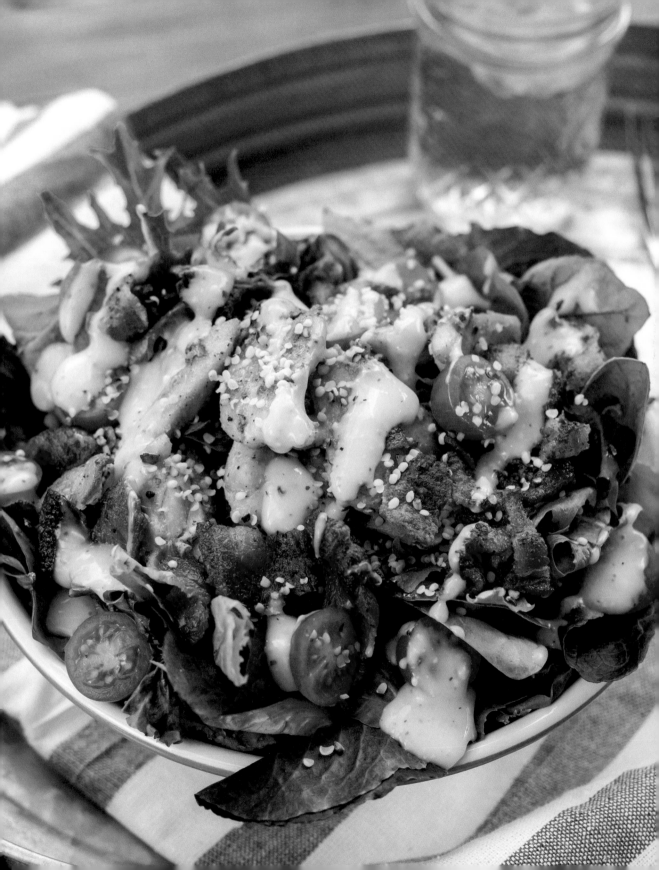

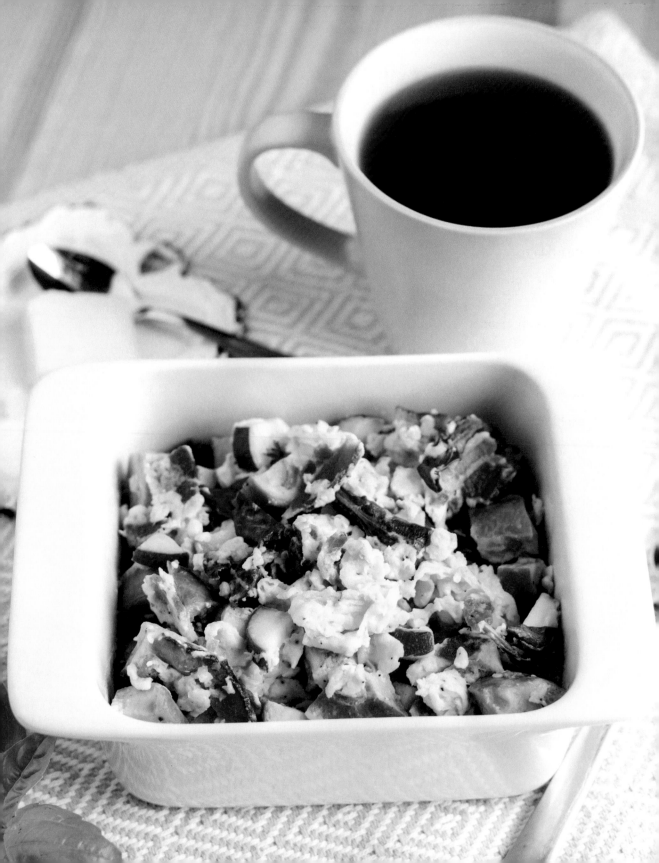

CHICKEN APPLE SAUSAGE SCRAMBLE

MAKES 1 SERVING

758 calories | 55g fat | 9g carbs | 52g protein

1 tablespoon ghee

4 eggs, beaten

1½ chicken apple sausages, sliced into bite-size pieces

2 slices bacon, cooked and crumbled

½ cup sliced zucchini

1 cup fresh spinach

Sea salt and pepper, to taste

Melt the ghee in a skillet, and add the eggs, chicken sausage, bacon, and vegetables. Season with salt and pepper to taste and scramble to desired doneness.

Serve and enjoy immediately.

CHICKEN CLUB WRAPS

MAKES 1 SERVING

592 calories | 48g fat | 8g carbs | 32g protein

3 ounces chicken breast, cooked and shredded

1½ tablespoons paleo mayo

Sea salt, to taste

Garlic powder, to taste

2 romaine lettuce leaves

4 slices of bacon, cooked

1 tablespoon paleo ranch

½ medium avocado, sliced

Toss the chicken in a small bowl with mayo, salt, and garlic powder.

Lay the lettuce leaves on a plate; divide the bacon between lettuce leaves. Add shredded chicken breast and drizzle with ranch. Top with avocado, sprinkle with sea salt, and enjoy immediately!

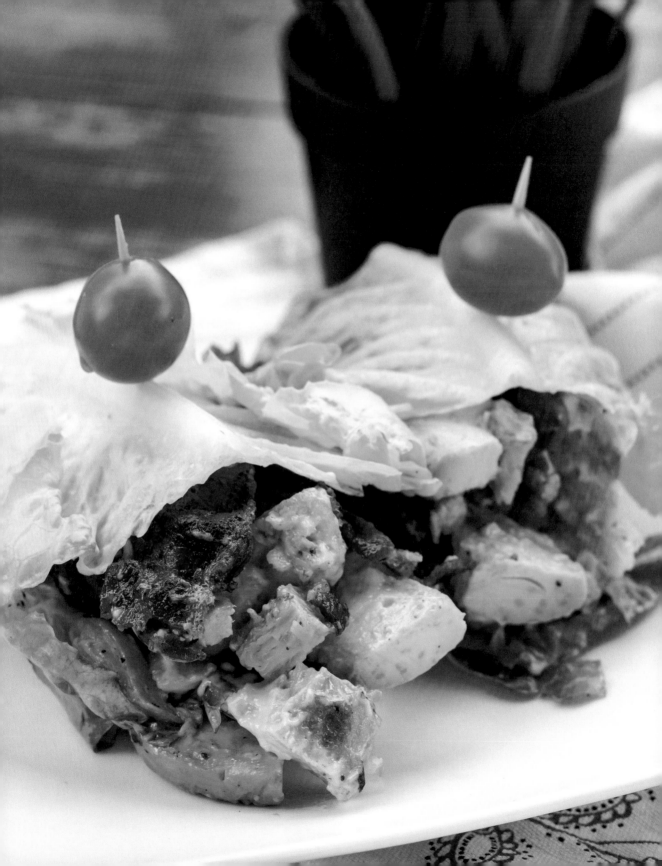

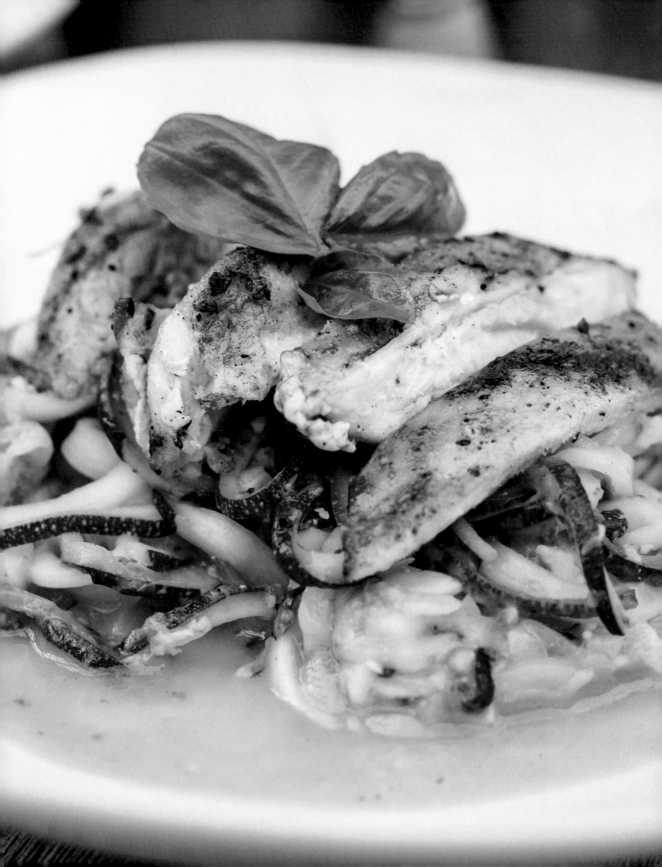

CHICKEN PESTO SALAD

MAKES 1 SERVING

522 calories | 45g fat | 7g carbs | 21g protein

1½ tablespoons olive oil

1 teaspoon minced garlic

6 ounces zucchini, spiralized (zoodles)

3 ounces boneless, skinless chicken thighs, cooked and sliced

3 tablespoons pesto

Drizzle the olive oil in a medium skillet, and sauté the minced garlic over medium-high heat until fragrant, about 2 minutes. Add the zoodles and continue to sauté until bright green and just soft, about 5 minutes. Remove from heat.

Add the chicken breast and pesto. Toss until well coated. Enjoy immediately!

CINNAMON PANCAKES
WITH BACON & EGGS

MAKES 1 SERVING

825 calories	71g fat	5g carbs	41g protein
Per pancake: 240 calories	22g fat	4g carbs	6g protein (1g net carbs)

FOR PANCAKES:

¼ teaspoon vanilla extract

¼ teaspoon almond extract

3 eggs

¼ cup ghee, melted

¼ cup coconut milk, from a can

2 tablespoons stevia or monk fruit sweetener

¼ cup coconut flour

¼ teaspoon sea salt

½ teaspoon baking powder

¼ teaspoon cinnamon

1 tablespoon whipped coconut cream

FOR BACON AND EGGS:

3 eggs

1½ tablespoons ghee

4 slices bacon, cooked

For the pancakes, in a blender combine the wet ingredients, except for the whipped coconut cream. In a small bowl combine the dry ingredients, and mix until well combined. Add the dry ingredients to the blender and mix until a batter forms. Allow the batter to rest 5 minutes; if it becomes too thick you may add water, 1 tablespoon at a time, to thin it out.

Heat a griddle to medium heat and spray it with nonstick cooking spray. Divide the batter into 4 large pancakes and cook until edges are set and golden brown, about 2 to 3 minutes. Flip and allow to cook another 2 minutes. (*Pancake recipe makes 4 servings.*)

Meanwhile, fry the eggs in 1 tablespoon of ghee to desired doneness. Serve 1 pancake topped with remaining ½ tablespoon of ghee, whipped coconut cream, and eggs and bacon on the side. Enjoy!

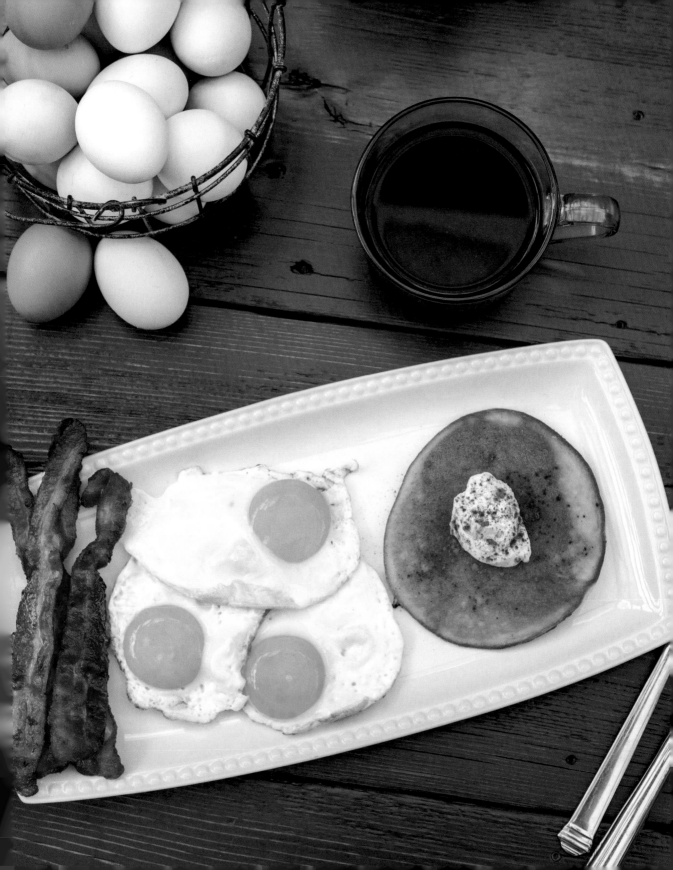

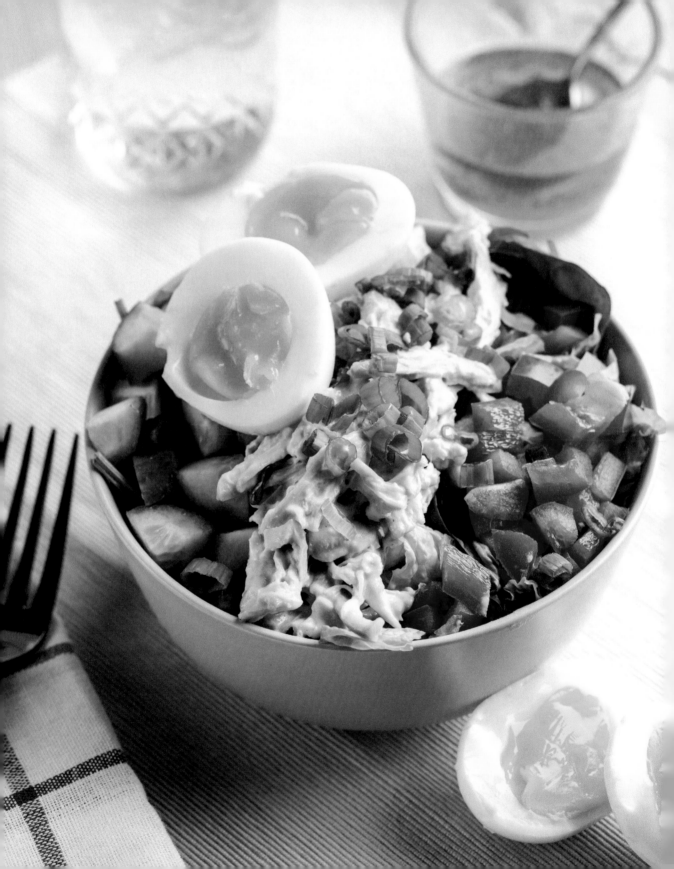

DIJON MUSTARD CHICKEN SALAD

MAKES 1 SERVING

831 calories | 54g fat | 12g carbs | 42g protein

3 cups spring salad mix

2 hard-boiled eggs, sliced

½ cup diced cucumbers

½ cup diced bell pepper

4 ounces cooked chicken breast, shredded

2 teaspoons Dijon mustard

1 tablespoon paleo mayo

Garlic powder, to taste

2 tablespoons avocado oil

1 tablespoon apple cider vinegar

Sea salt and pepper, to taste

2 spring onions, chopped

Layer the spring salad, eggs, cucumbers, and bell pepper in a large bowl

Toss the chicken with Dijon mustard, paleo mayo, and garlic powder in a small bowl until well coated. Place the chicken on top of the salad.

Combine the avocado oil, vinegar, salt, and pepper in a separate small bowl. Drizzle over the salad, sprinkle with spring onions, and enjoy!

DREW'S B.A.E.

526 calories | 41g fat | 8g carbs | 30g protein

3 slices bacon

3 eggs

Sea salt and pepper, to taste

½ tablespoon ghee

1 cup fresh spinach

½ medium avocado

Fry the bacon to desired texture in a skillet. Once cooked, remove it from skillet and set it aside.

Break the eggs into a small bowl and whisk together, then scramble them in the skillet, seasoning with sea salt and pepper to taste.

While the eggs are scrambling, melt the ghee over medium heat in a small pan. Add the spinach and sauté until it's wilted.

Add the spinach to the eggs as they finish cooking and mix together. Enjoy with bacon and avocado, seasoned with sea salt, on the side.

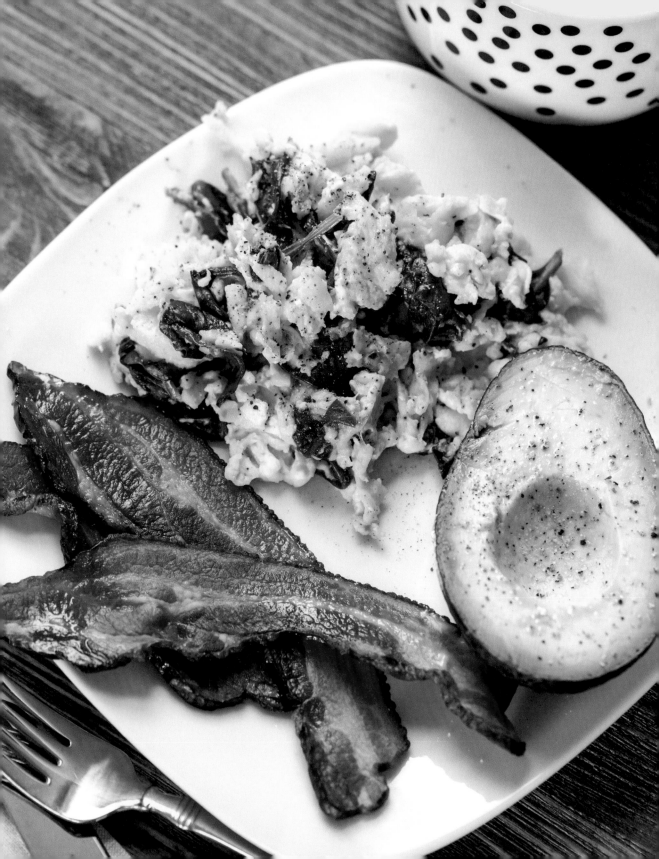

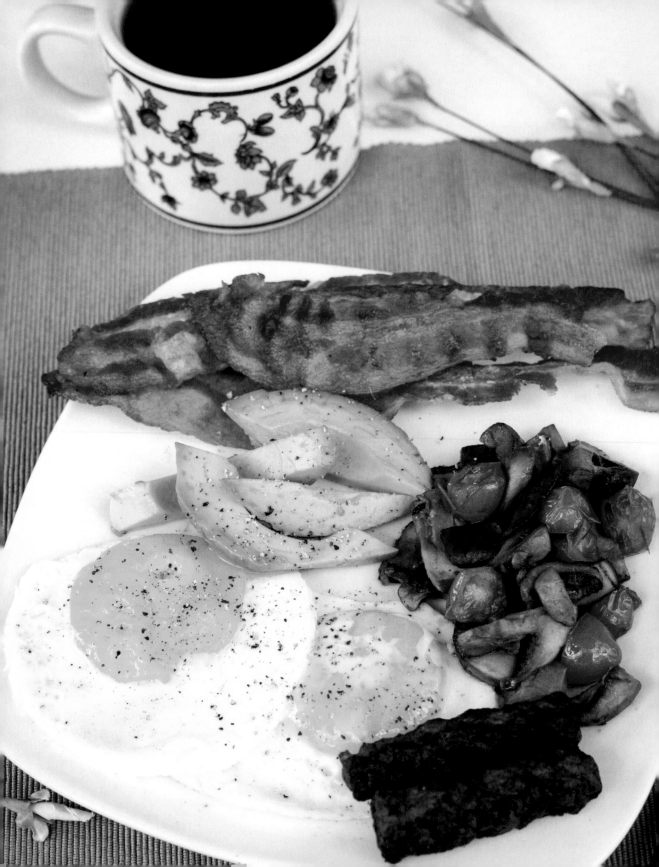

ENGLISH BREAKFAST PLATE

MAKES 1 SERVING

651 calories | 53g fat | 13g carbs | 30g protein

1 tablespoon ghee

2 eggs

Sea salt and pepper, to taste

5 cherry tomatoes, halved

½ cup mushrooms

3 slices bacon, cooked

½ medium avocado

2 breakfast sausage links, cooked

Melt ½ tablespoon of the ghee over medium heat in a medium skillet. Break the eggs in the preheated pan and season to taste. Fry the eggs to desired doneness and set aside.

Melt the remaining ghee in the same skillet, add the tomatoes and mushrooms, and season to taste. Sauté until the mushrooms and tomatoes soften, about 5 to 7 minutes.

Place the mushroom mixture on a plate with the eggs, bacon, avocado, and sausage on the side! Enjoy!

GREEK STEAK SALAD

MAKES 1 SERVING

543 calories | 42g fat | 9g carbs | 33g protein

2 cups romaine salad mix

1 ounce kalamata olives, sliced

½ cup chopped cucumbers

6 ounces rib eye steak, cooked and sliced in strips

2 tablespoons paleo Greek vinaigrette dressing

Cumin, to taste

Paprika, to taste

Layer the romaine salad mix, olives, and cucumbers in a bowl. Top with the steak and drizzle the dressing over the top. Season with cumin and paprika as desired. Enjoy!

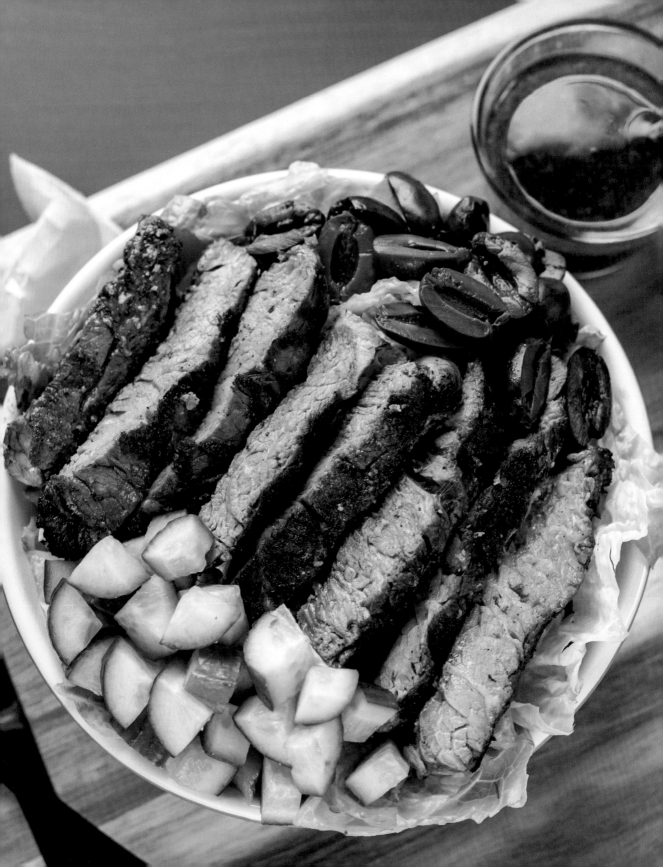

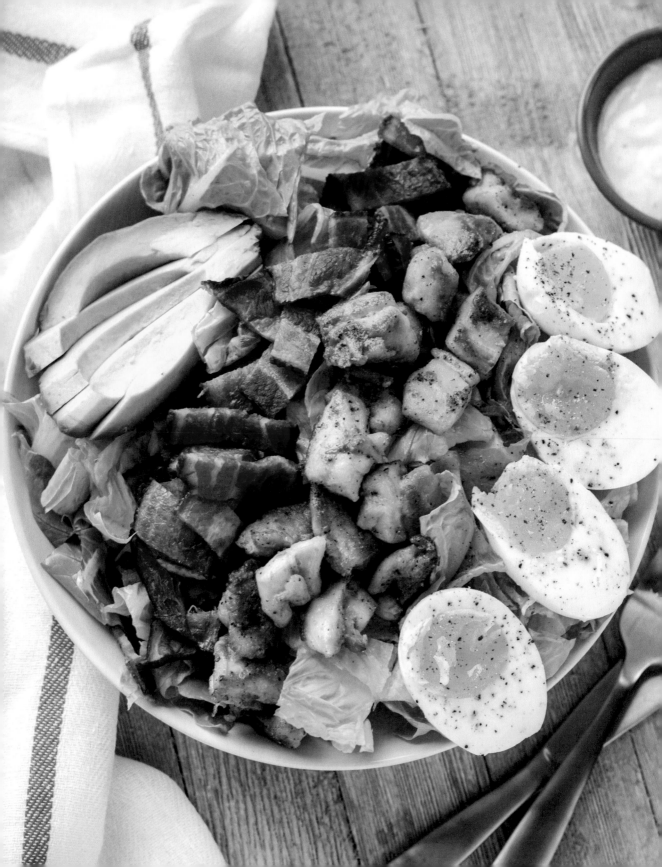

KETO COBB SALAD

MAKES 1 SERVING

721 calories | 61g fat | 10g carbs | 35g protein

1 tablespoon avocado oil

2 ounces boneless, skinless chicken thighs, chopped

Sea salt and pepper, to taste

3 cups romaine salad mix

2 hard-boiled eggs, sliced

3 slices bacon, cooked and crumbled

⅓ medium avocado, sliced

2 tablespoons paleo ranch dressing

Drizzle the avocado oil in a skillet and add the chicken thighs, sea salt, and pepper. Sauté over medium heat until cooked through and no longer pink, about 8 to 10 minutes.

Meanwhile, layer the salad mix, sliced hard-boiled eggs, bacon, and avocado in a large bowl.

Top the salad with the cooked chicken thighs and drizzle ranch over the salad. Enjoy!

KETO-RITO

845 calories | 71g fat | 5g carbs | 46g protein

3 ounces ground breakfast sausage

⅓ cup diced mushrooms

4 eggs

1 tablespoon ghee

Sea salt and pepper, to taste

2 tablespoons guacamole

2 slices bacon, cooked and diced

Hot sauce, to taste

Heat a medium skillet over medium heat, and add the ground breakfast sausage and mushrooms. Sauté until the sausage is crumbled and cooked through, and the mushrooms are soft. Set aside.

Beat 2 eggs in a small bowl until well combined. Melt ½ tablespoon of ghee in the same skillet; add the eggs and season with salt and pepper to taste. Allow the eggs to fry; do not scramble, as this will be your "tortilla." Allow the edges to begin to set, about 2 to 3 minutes. Once the edges and most of the center are set, flip the eggs, allow them to cook another minute, and then remove from heat. Repeat with remaining eggs and ghee.

Spread ½ tablespoon of the guacamole in each "tortilla," add the sausage and mushroom mixture, and sprinkle bacon down the middle of the "tortilla."

Top with the remaining guacamole and hot sauce. Roll up and enjoy!

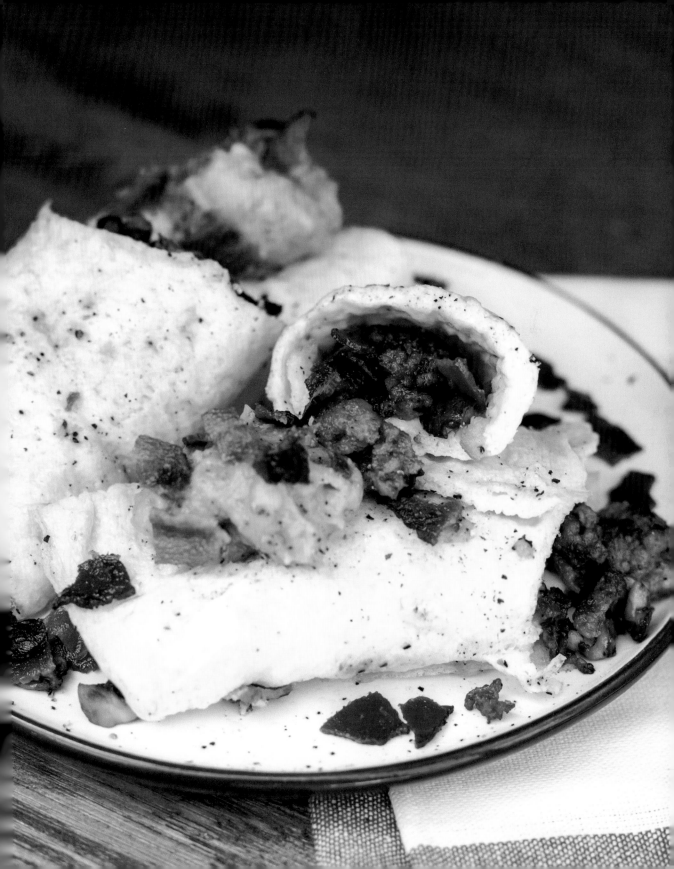

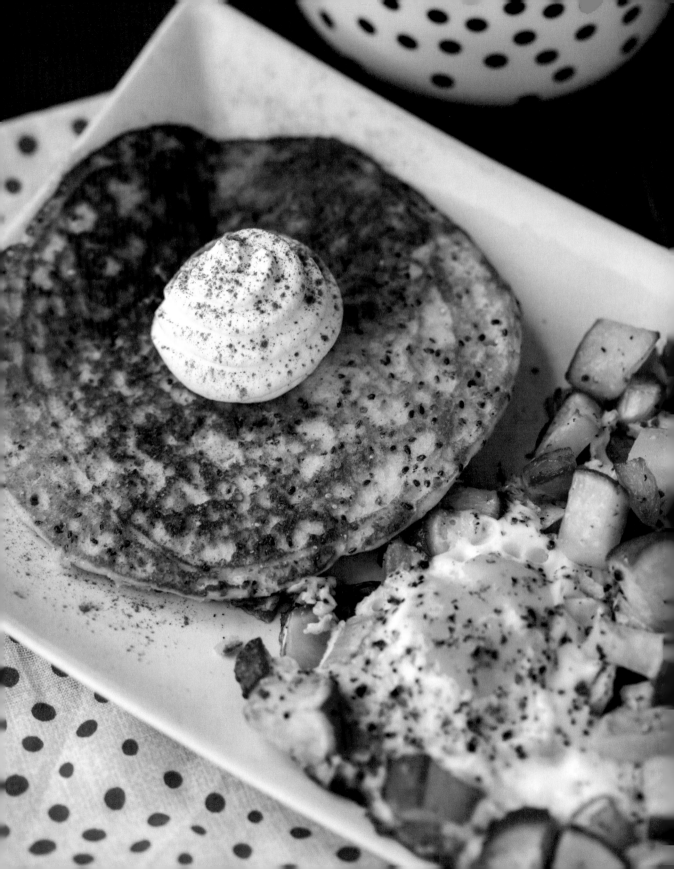

LEMON CHIA PANCAKES
WITH RADISH HASH & POACHED EGGS

MAKES 1 SERVING

700 calories	61g fat	19g carbs	21g protein	
Per pancake: 257 calories	23g fat	6g carbs	6g protein (2g net carbs)	

FOR PANCAKES:

¼ cup coconut milk, from a can

2 tablespoons lemon juice

2 tablespoons stevia or monk fruit sweetener

¼ teaspoon vanilla extract

¼ teaspoon almond extract

3 eggs

¼ cup ghee, melted

¼ cup coconut flour

1 tablespoon chia seeds

¼ teaspoon sea salt

½ teaspoon baking powder

2 tablespoons whipped coconut cream

FOR HASH:

1½ tablespoons avocado oil

1½ cups chopped radishes

¼ cup chopped onion

¼ teaspoon minced garlic

Sea salt and pepper, to taste

2 eggs

2 tablespoons chopped green onion

For the pancakes, combine the wet ingredients in a blender, except for the whipped coconut cream. Combine the dry ingredients in a small bowl, except for the chia seeds; mix until well combined. Add the dry ingredients to the blender and mix until a batter forms. Pour the batter into a bowl and fold in the chia seeds. Allow the batter to rest for 5 minutes; if the batter becomes too thick you may add water, 1 tablespoon at a time, to thin it out.

Heat a griddle to medium heat and spray with nonstick cooking spray. Divide batter into 4 large pancakes and cook until edges are set and golden brown, about 2 to 3 minutes. Then flip them and allow to cook another 2 minutes. (*Pancake recipe makes 4 servings.*)

While the pancakes are cooking, add 1 tablespoon of avocado oil to a skillet, and add radishes, onion, and garlic. Season with sea salt and pepper. Sauté over medium heat until the radishes are browned and the onion is translucent, about 5 to 8 minutes.

Create 2 small wells in the hash, divide the remaining oil between the two wells, and crack an egg into each well. Season the eggs with the sea salt and pepper to taste. Cover the hash with a lid and allow the eggs to poach, about 3 to 5 minutes or until eggs are white and cooked to desired doneness. Sprinkle green onion on top.

Enjoy 1 pancake, topped with whipped coconut cream, with radish hash on the side!

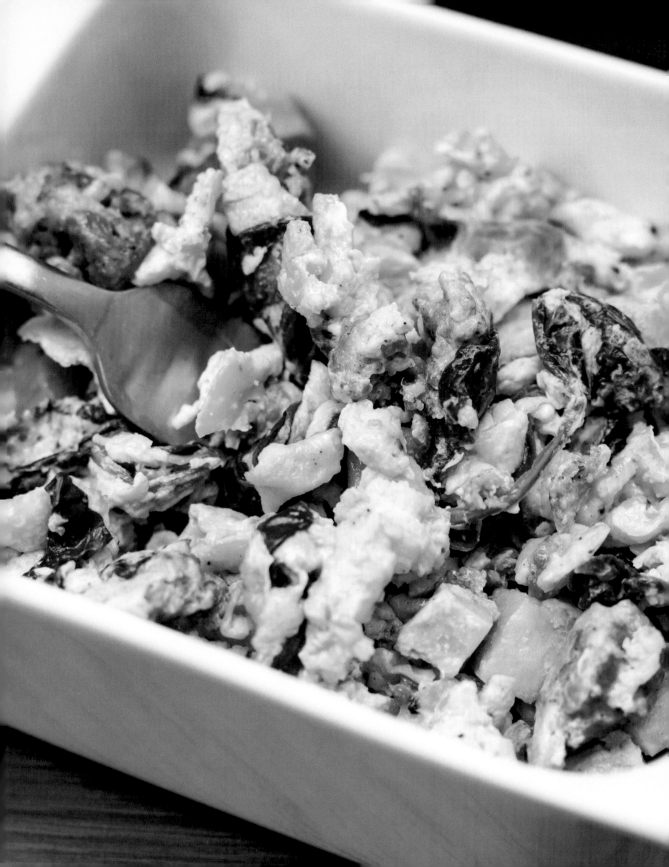

MEAT LOVERS' SCRAMBLE

MAKES 1 SERVING

624 calories | 49g fat | 4g carbs | 41g protein

4 eggs

Sea salt and pepper, to taste

1 tablespoon ghee

1½ ounces diced ham

1½ ounces ground pork sausage, cooked

1 to 2 handfuls fresh spinach

No-sugar-added hot sauce (optional)

Beat the eggs with the seasonings in a small bowl until mixed well.

Heat the ghee in a medium skillet until melted, swirling it around until it coats the bottom of the pan.

Add the eggs, ham, sausage, and spinach. Scramble until cooked as desired.

Serve the eggs with the hot sauce on top and enjoy!

SAUSAGE FRITTATA & FRIED RADISHES

MAKES 1 SERVING

663 calories | 54g fat | 9g carbs | 36g protein

1 tablespoon ghee

3 eggs

Sea salt and pepper, to taste

½ cup sliced mushrooms

1 cup chopped spinach

3 ounces ground pork sausage, cooked

1 cup chopped radishes

Preheat the oven to 400 degrees Fahrenheit. Melt ½ tablespoon of ghee in a small cast-iron skillet, and swirl it around to evenly coat the bottom to avoid sticking. Beat the eggs together in a small bowl, seasoning with sea salt and pepper.

Pour the eggs into the skillet, then sprinkle the mushrooms over the top of the eggs, followed by spinach and sausage.

Place the skillet in the preheated oven and bake for 8 to 10 minutes, or until the frittata is set. Once cooked, remove it from the oven and allow it to cool.

Meanwhile, place the remaining ghee in a skillet with the radishes. Season with sea salt and pepper. Sauté until browned and just soft, about 6 to 8 minutes. Enjoy the frittata with radishes on the side.

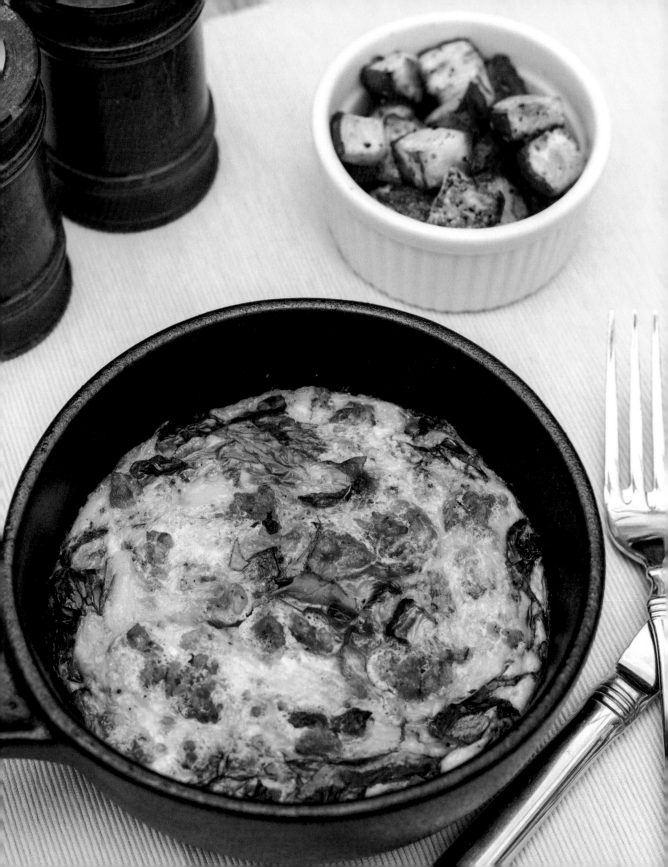

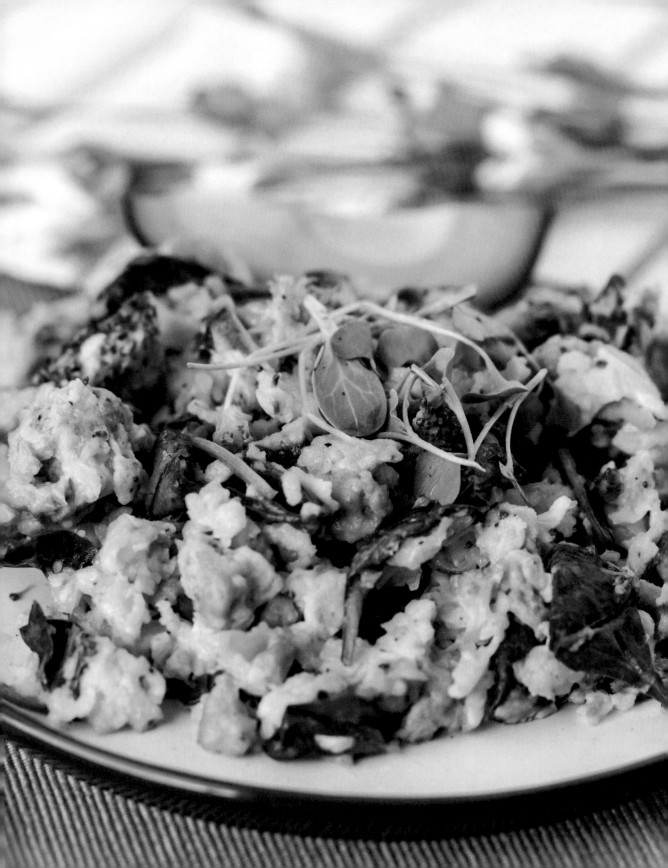

SAUSAGE SCRAMBLE

MAKES 1 SERVING

699 calories | 58g fat | 7g carbs | 36g protein

1 tablespoon avocado oil

3 eggs, beaten

3 ounces ground pork sausage, cooked

⅓ cup chopped broccoli

1 cup fresh spinach

Sea salt and pepper, to taste

¼ medium avocado, sliced

Put the avocado oil in a medium skillet over medium heat, and swirl it around to grease the skillet.

Once the oil is sizzling, add in remaining ingredients, except avocado, and scramble until eggs are cooked through and spinach is wilted.

Place on a plate and top with sliced avocado. Enjoy immediately!

SAVORY SAUSAGE OPEN-FACE SANDWICH

MAKES 1 SERVING

831 calories | 69g fat | 15g carbs | 36g protein

FOR THE BISCUIT:

3 tablespoons coconut flour

1 egg

1½ tablespoons ghee

½ teaspoon baking powder

¼ teaspoon sea salt

¼ teaspoon garlic powder

FOR THE FIXINGS:

2½ ounces ground pork sausage

2 eggs

½ tablespoon ghee

1 cup fresh spinach

Spray a microwave-safe mug with nonstick cooking spray. Add the coconut flour, egg, ghee, baking powder, seasonings, and 1 tablespoon water. Mix until well combined. Place in a microwave for 1 minute 45 seconds, or until set. Allow it to cool before removing it.

Meanwhile, form pork sausage into two small patties. Fry them in a skillet over medium heat until cooked through, about 3 minutes on each side. Set them aside once cooked through.

Fry the eggs in sausage grease to desired doneness, and set them aside.

Melt the ghee in the same skillet and sauté the spinach until it is wilted, about 2 to 3 minutes.

Remove the biscuit from the mug and cut it in half. Top each slice with spinach, sausage, and egg. Enjoy immediately!

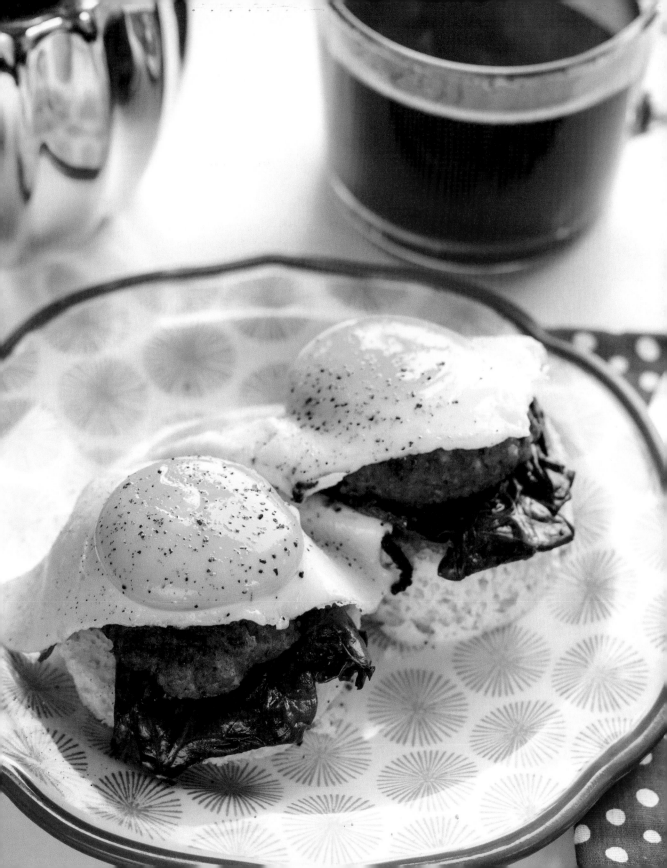

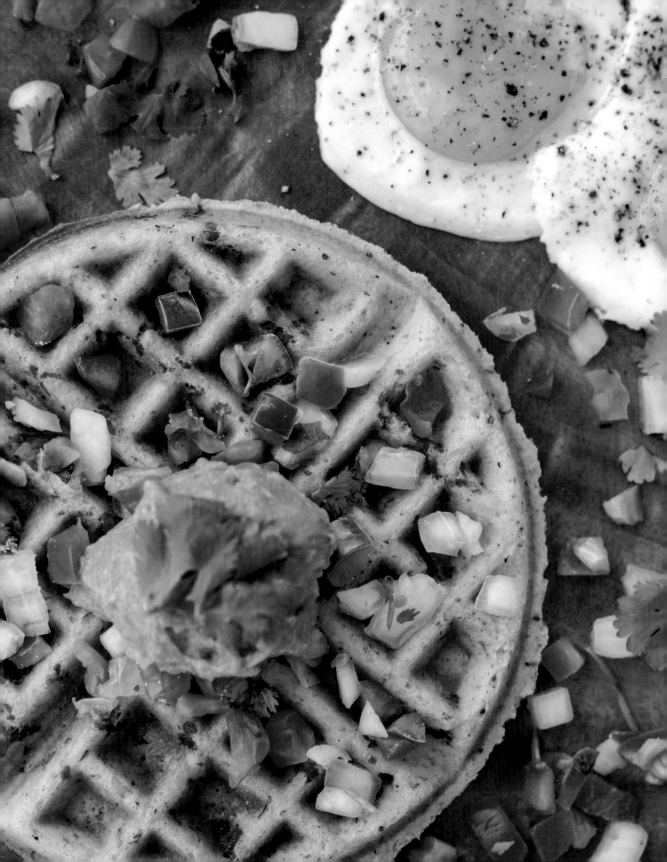

SAVORY WAFFLES WITH EGGS & PICO

MAKES 2 WAFFLES (1 waffle per serving) | 1 SERVING EGGS & PICO

746 calories | 65g fat | 10g carbs | 33g protein

For a single waffle: 405 calories | 35g fat | 6g carbs | 20g protein

FOR THE WAFFLES:

3 eggs

2 tablespoons ghee, melted

¼ teaspoon sea salt

¼ teaspoon garlic powder

½ teaspoon Italian seasoning

Pinch of onion powder

¼ teaspoon baking powder

3 tablespoons coconut flour

3 ounces ground pork breakfast sausage, cooked and crumbled

FOR THE EGGS AND PICO:

1 tablespoon ghee

2 eggs

2 tablespoons guacamole

2 tablespoons pico de gallo

For the waffles, combine the eggs and melted ghee in a blender or food processor. Blend them until thoroughly combined. Then add the seasonings and baking powder, and mix. Add the coconut flour and mix until the batter is smooth. Fold in the cooked sausage and allow the batter to rest.

Heat a Belgian waffle iron and spray it with nonstick cooking spray. Pour half the batter into the preheated waffle iron, and cook according to the waffle iron manufacturer's instructions. The recipe makes 2 waffles, so you can save the leftovers for another day or share with family and friends.

Meanwhile, as the waffles are cooking, melt the remaining ghee in a skillet over medium heat. Fry the eggs to desired doneness.

Place the eggs and 1 waffle on a plate. Top the waffle with guacamole and pico de gallo, and enjoy!

SHREDDED PORK SALAD

MAKES 1 SERVING

607 calories | 50g fat | 11g carbs | 30g protein

2 cups romaine salad mix

3 slices bacon

3 ounces cooked pulled pork butt

½ avocado, sliced

2 tablespoons paleo ranch dressing

Layer the romaine salad mix, bacon, and pulled pork in a bowl.

Top with the avocado, drizzle the paleo ranch dressing over the salad, and enjoy!

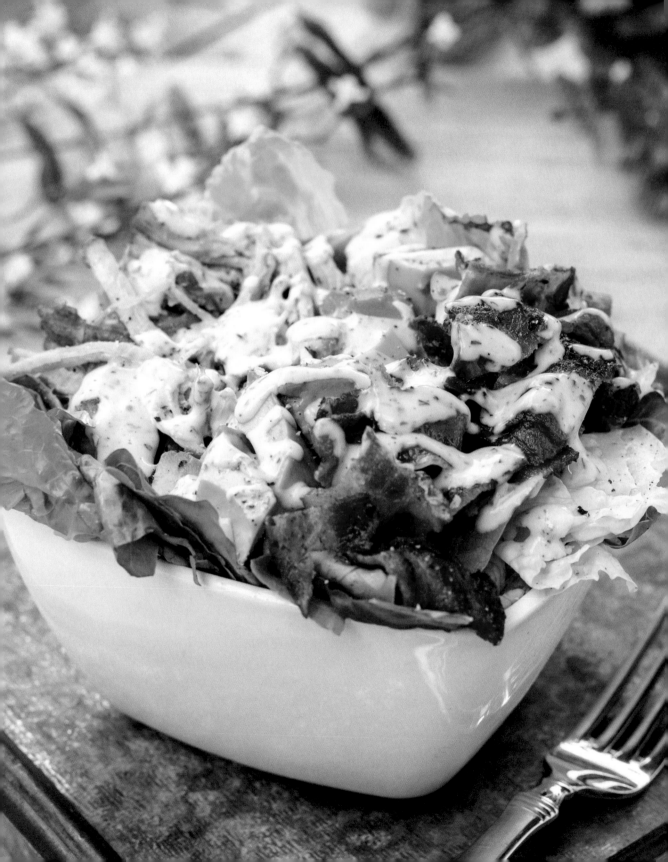

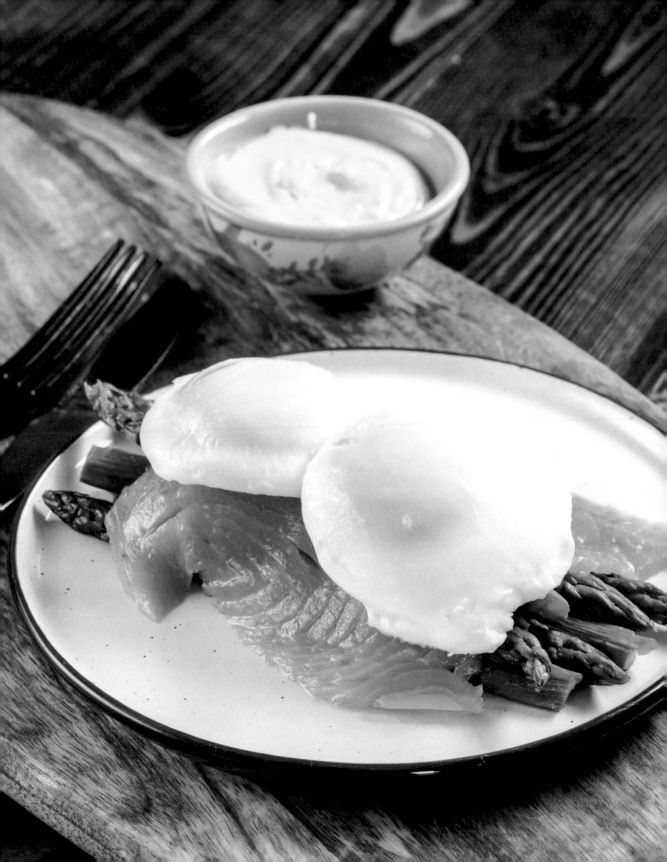

SMOKED SALMON & POACHED EGGS
with HOLLANDAISE SAUCE

MAKES 1 SERVING

571 calories | 46g fat | 6g carbs | 36g protein

2 eggs

1 cup asparagus

1 tablespoon avocado oil

Sea salt, to taste

3 ounces smoked salmon

¹⁄₁₀ serving Hollandaise sauce (measure out 10 servings)

FOR THE SAUCE:

3 egg yolks

½ cup ghee

Sea salt, to taste

Dash of cayenne

Add about 4 to 6 inches of water to a pot, just enough so that it will cover the eggs. Allow it to heat to 180 degrees Fahrenheit.

Crack the eggs into small ramekins. Once the water reaches the desired temperature, dip the ramekins into the water and slowly pour the eggs out into the water. (This helps keep the eggs together.) Allow to simmer about 5 to 6 minutes, until the whites are solid and cooked through.

Remove the eggs from the water using a slotted spoon. Place them on a napkin to remove excess water.

Meanwhile, sauté the asparagus in avocado oil in a skillet. Season it with sea salt, and continue sautéing until just soft and bright green.

Once the asparagus is cooked, place it on a plate, and top it with smoked salmon and poached eggs. Drizzle with Hollandaise sauce and enjoy!

INSTRUCTIONS FOR SAUCE:

Add the egg yolks to a wide-mouth jar that is just big enough for an immersion blender to fit in snugly.

Preheat a small frying pan over medium heat. Add the ghee and allow it to melt. Continue heating it until it begins to bubble and stops foaming.

Add the hot ghee to the jar, slowly, as you turn on the immersion blender. Then pour slightly faster as the Hollandaise begins to emulsify.

Once the sauce is nice and thick, add the seasonings, then allow the sauce to sit in the jar while you plate the rest of the dish. Hollandaise sauce does not refrigerate or keep well, so enjoy it as soon as possible!

SMOKED SALMON WEDGE SALAD

MAKES 1 SERVING

692 calories | 55g fat | 11g carbs | 36g protein

½ small head iceberg lettuce

3½ ounces smoked salmon

1 hard-boiled egg, sliced

2 slices bacon, cooked and crumbled

¼ medium avocado, sliced

FOR THE DRESSING:

1 tablespoon paleo mayo

1 tablespoon avocado oil

1 teaspoon Dijon mustard

Apple cider vinegar, to taste

Sea salt and pepper, to taste

Whisk together all the ingredients for the dressing in a small bowl and set it aside.

Cut the iceberg lettuce into 3 to 4 wedges. Top with smoked salmon and hard-boiled egg, and sprinkle with crumbled bacon and avocado.

Drizzle the wedge salad with the dressing and enjoy.

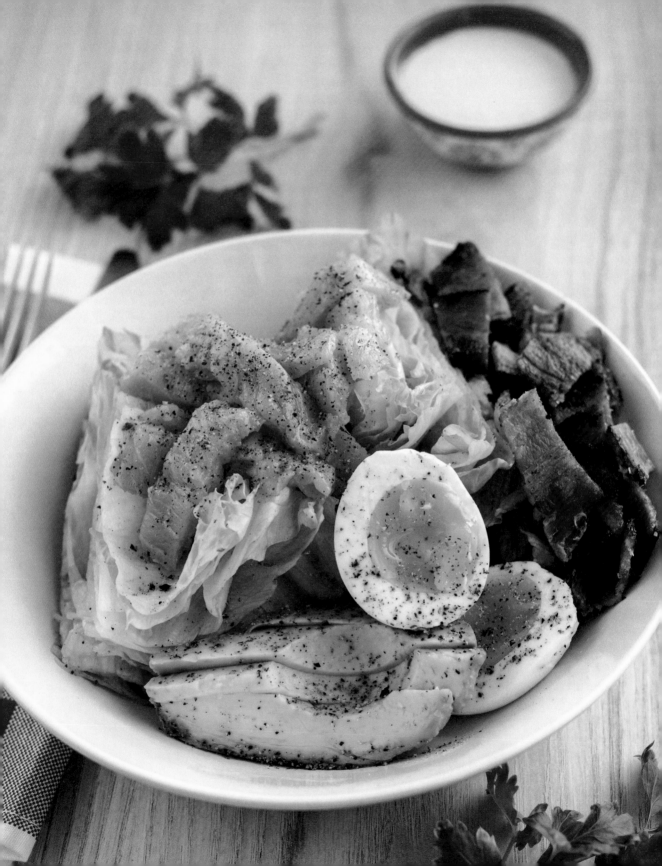

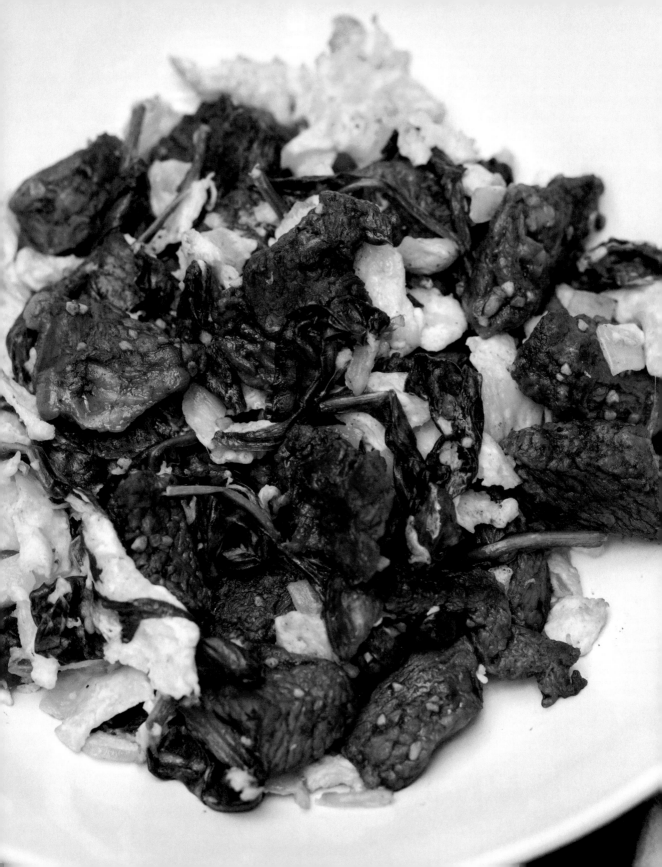

STEAK & EGGS BREAKFAST SCRAMBLE

MAKES 1 SERVING

633 calories | 51g fat | 6g carbs | 38g protein

4 ounce rib eye steak

Sea salt and pepper, to taste

Garlic powder, to taste

Paprika, to taste

1 tablespoon ghee

½ cup sliced onion

2 eggs

2 cups spinach

Preheat a grill to medium heat, and season the steak with the salt, pepper, and garlic powder to taste on both sides, using your fingers to rub it in. Grill the steak to desired doneness.

Meanwhile, melt ¼ tablespoon of ghee in a skillet and add the onion. Sauté until the onion is translucent.

Melt the remaining ghee in the same skillet and add the eggs and spinach. Scramble until the eggs are cooked through and the spinach is wilted.

Serve the steak with eggs and enjoy!

STEAK FAJITA SALAD

MAKES 1 SERVING

575 calories | 41g fat | 12g carbs | 38g protein

1 tablespoon ghee

6 ounces flank steak, sliced

½ teaspoon no-sugar-added taco seasoning

¼ cup sliced onion

½ green bell pepper, sliced

2 cups romaine salad mix

2 tablespoons paleo ranch dressing

1 green onion stalk, chopped

Melt ¼ tablespoon of ghee in a skillet over high heat, and allow it to heat for 1 minute. Season the steak with no-sugar-added taco seasoning. Add the steak to the skillet, cook it to desired doneness, and then set it aside.

Melt the remaining ghee in the same pan, add the onion and pepper, and sauté until just soft.

Layer the romaine salad mix, pepper and onion mixture, and steak in a large bowl. Drizzle the salad with ranch dressing and sprinkle with the green onions. Enjoy!

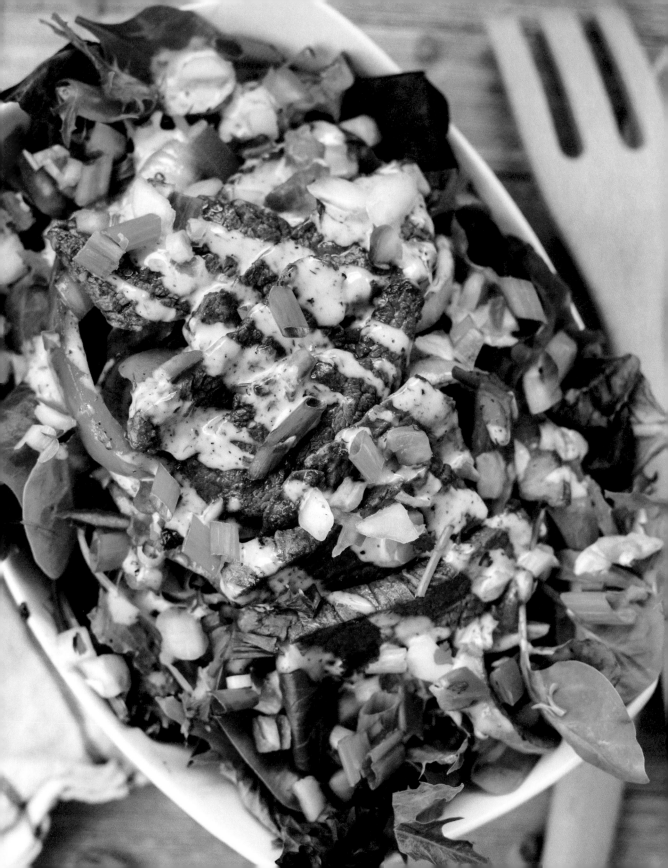

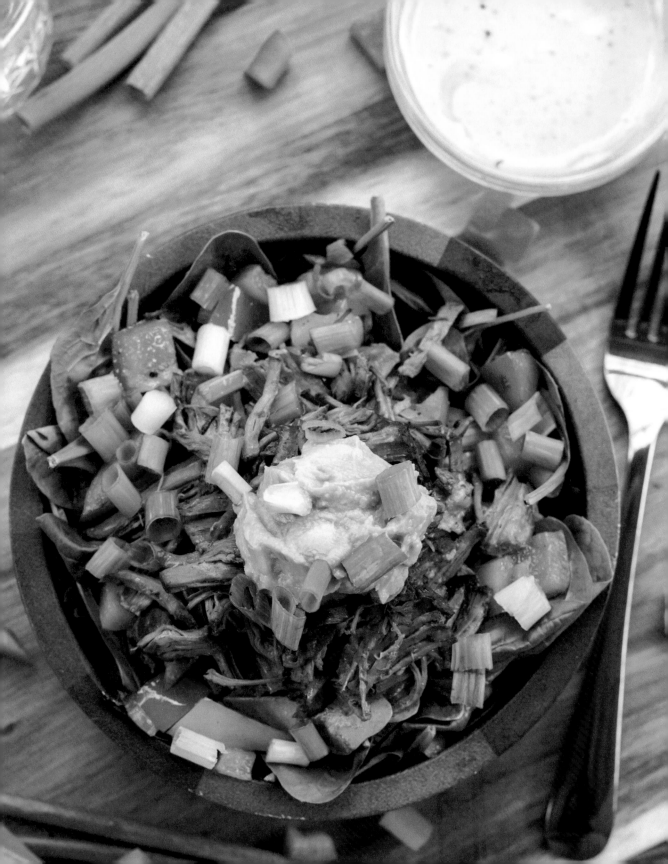

TACO SALAD & CHIPOTLE DRESSING

MAKES 1 SERVING

705 calories | 61g fat | 11g carbs | 31g protein

4 ounces cooked roast beef, shredded

1 tablespoon avocado oil

1 teaspoon no-sugar-added taco seasoning

¼ cup sliced onion

¼ cup sliced bell pepper

Sea salt and pepper, to taste

3 cups spinach

1 green onion, chopped

1 tablespoon guacamole

FOR THE CHIPOTLE DRESSING:

2 tablespoons paleo mayo

1 tablespoon apple cider vinegar

1 teaspoon hot sauce

½ teaspoon chipotle seasoning

Toss the shredded beef with 1/4 tablespoon of avocado oil and taco seasoning until well coated. Set it aside.

Add the remaining avocado oil, onion, pepper, and seasonings to a skillet. Sauté until just soft, about 5 to 6 minutes.

For the dressing, mix the paleo mayo, vinegar, hot sauce, and chipotle seasoning in a small bowl.

Layer the spinach, peppers, onions, and beef in a bowl. Top with the green onion and guacamole. Drizzle with chipotle dressing, and enjoy!

KETO
DINNER

BACON BISON BURGER

MAKES 1 SERVING

692 calories | 52g fat | 6g carbs | 49g protein

6 ounces ground bison

Garlic powder, to taste

Cumin, to taste

Paprika, to taste

1 cup broccolini

1 tablespoon olive oil

Sea salt, to taste

1 large leaf romaine

1 tablespoon chipotle paleo mayo

2 slices bacon, cooked

1 egg, fried

Combine the ground bison and seasonings in a large bowl. Use your hands to form the ground bison into a burger patty.

Preheat the grill to medium heat, and cook the burger to desired doneness.

Meanwhile, preheat the oven to 375 degrees, and toss the broccolini with olive oil and sea salt. Bake on a baking sheet for 15 minutes.

Place the burger patty on lettuce, and top with chipotle mayo, 2 slices of bacon, and fried egg. Enjoy with broccolini on the side immediately!

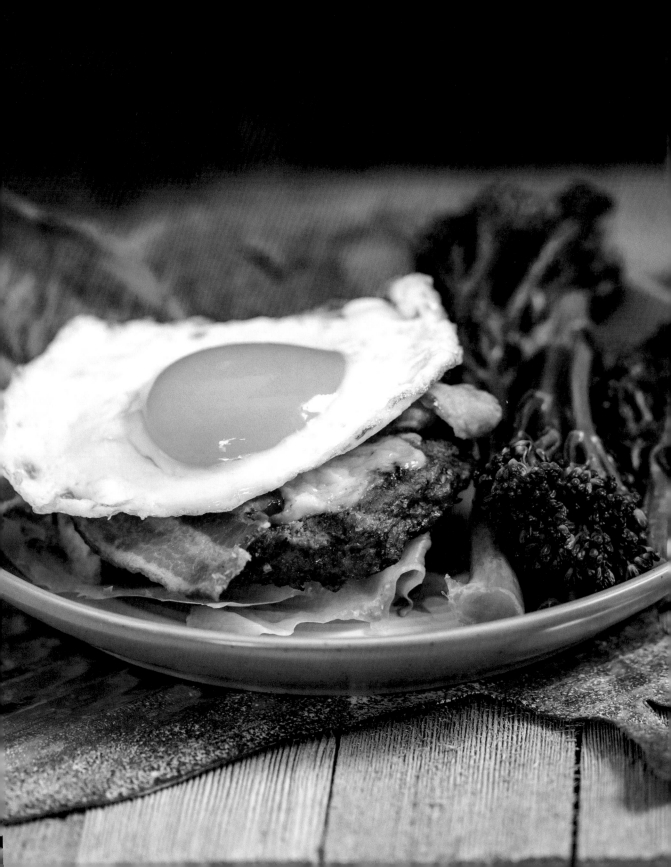

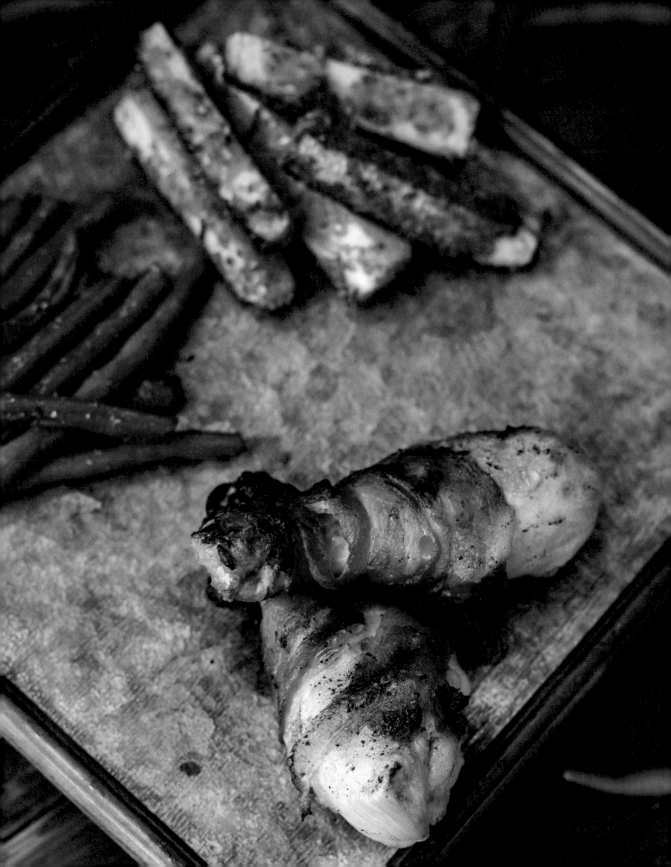

BACON-WRAPPED CHICKEN DRUMSTICK & FRIED ZUCCHINI

MAKES 1 SERVING

757 calories | 62g fat | 11g carbs | 42g protein

4-ounce chicken drumstick

Sea salt and pepper, to taste

2 slices bacon

1 medium zucchini

1 egg

½ ounce pork rinds, crushed fine

1 tablespoon unsweetened shredded coconut

Stevia, to taste

Pinch of dried parsley

2 tablespoons coconut oil

½ cup green beans

½ tablespoon avocado oil

Preheat grill to medium heat.

Pat the drumstick dry with a paper towel, and season with sea salt and pepper to taste on all sides. Wrap the bacon slices around the drumstick, tucking the ends so they do not unravel while cooking.

Place the drumstick on the grill and cook for 30 to 35 minutes, flipping every 5 to 7 minutes, or until it reaches an internal temperature of 185 degrees Fahrenheit.

Meanwhile, as the drumstick is cooking, slice the zucchini into spears and set them aside. Beat the egg in a medium bowl until thoroughly combined. In another bowl mix together the pork rinds, shredded coconut, and seasonings.

Melt the coconut oil over high heat in a large pan.

Dip the zucchini into the egg wash, and then roll in the pork rind mixture. Fry in heated coconut oil until edges are golden brown, about 2 minutes; then flip and cook another 1 to 2 minutes.

While frying, steam the green beans, and once steamed, toss in the avocado oil and season with salt and pepper.

Enjoy the drumstick with the green beans and fried zucchini on the side!

BACON-WRAPPED SALMON

MAKES 1 SERVING

846 calories | 69g fat | 10g carbs | 40g protein

2 tablespoons avocado oil

4-ounce wild-caught salmon fillet

Paprika, to taste

Chili powder, to taste

2 slices bacon

1½ cups chopped cauliflower

Sea salt and pepper, to taste

2 cups mixed greens

2 tablespoons paleo Greek vinaigrette

8 pitted black olives

Preheat oven to 375 degrees Fahrenheit. Line a baking sheet with foil, spray with nonstick cooking spray, and set aside.

Rub ½ tablespoon of avocado oil on both sides of the salmon. Season the fillet with paprika and chili powder to taste, and then wrap it with bacon.

Heat ½ tablespoon of avocado oil in a pan over medium-high heat. Fry the salmon on each side until it is golden brown, about 2 minutes per side.

Remove the salmon from the heat and place it on a baking sheet. Bake it in the preheated oven until cooked through, about 8 to 10 minutes, or until it reaches an internal temperature of 145 degrees Fahrenheit.

Meanwhile, as the salmon cooks, sauté the cauliflower in the remaining avocado oil, and season with salt and pepper. Sauté until soft, about 6 to 8 minutes.

Enjoy the salmon with salad drizzled with dressing, olives, and cauliflower on the side!

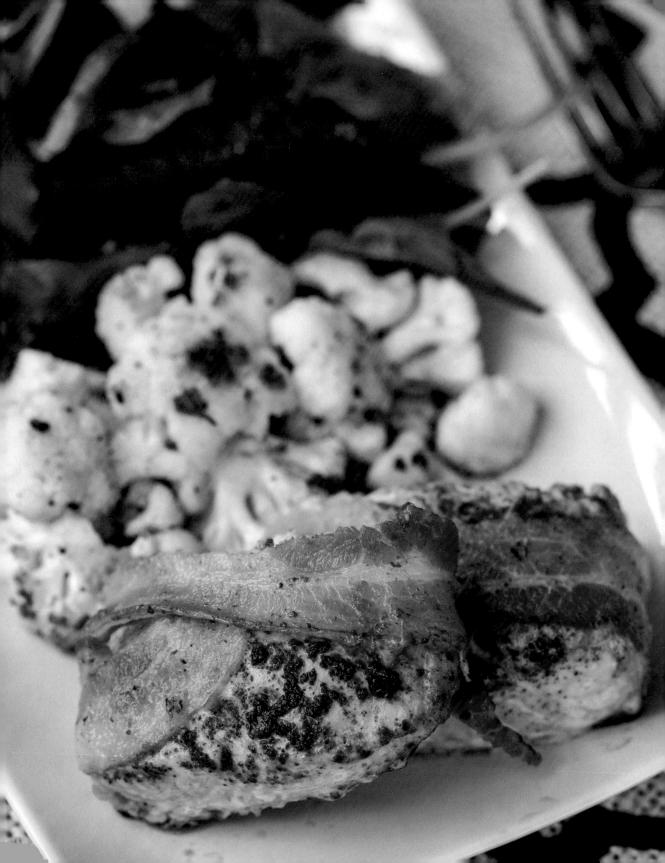

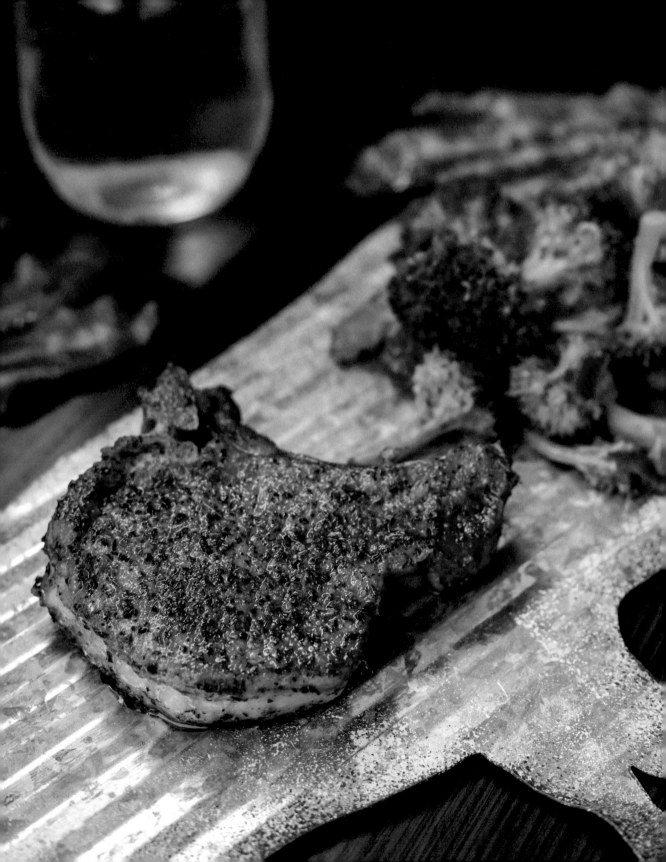

BAKED RANCH PORK CHOPS
WITH BACON BROCCOLI

MAKES 1 SERVING

809 calories | 60g fat | 9g carbs | 57g protein

6-ounce bone-in pork chop

Sea salt and pepper, to taste

½ teaspoon Italian seasoning

¼ teaspoon paprika

1½ tablespoons paleo ranch

1½ tablespoons ghee

2 cups chopped broccoli

½ teaspoon minced garlic

2 slices bacon, chopped

Preheat oven to 350 degrees Fahrenheit. Spray a small baking dish with nonstick cooking spray.

Season both sides of pork chop with salt and pepper. Place it in the baking dish, and sprinkle Italian seasoning and paprika over the top of the pork chop. Top with paleo ranch, and then pour ¼ cup of water into the bottom of the baking dish.

Cover the baking dish with foil, tightly pinching the edges closed. Bake for 45 minutes, remove the foil, and then continue baking for 15 to 20 minutes, or until pork reaches an internal temperature of 160 degrees.

Meanwhile, melt the ghee over medium heat in a skillet. Add the broccoli, minced garlic, and bacon, and season with sea salt to taste. Toss until well coated, and cook until the broccoli is bright green and the bacon is cooked through, about 5 to 6 minutes.

Enjoy the pork chop with broccoli on the side.

BEEF & BROCCOLI STIR-FRY

MAKES 1 SERVING

635 calories | 50g fat | 10g carbs | 35g protein

6 ounces flat iron steak, sliced

2 tablespoons avocado oil

½ teaspoon sesame oil

Sea salt and pepper, to taste

Ground ginger, to taste

½ cup broccoli

1 cup cauliflower rice

2 teaspoons coconut aminos

1 teaspoon minced garlic

Stir-fry the steak in 1 tablespoon of avocado oil and sesame oil in a large skillet over medium heat. Season with sea salt, pepper, and ginger to taste. Cook until the steak reaches desired doneness, then remove it from the pan and set it aside.

Add in the broccoli and remaining avocado oil, stir-frying until it is bright green and just tender, about 4 to 5 minutes.

Add in the cauliflower rice, coconut aminos, garlic, and more ginger to taste. Stir-fry until the cauliflower just begins to color, about 3 minutes. Add in the beef, thoroughly combine for 1 minute, and then remove from heat.

Enjoy immediately.

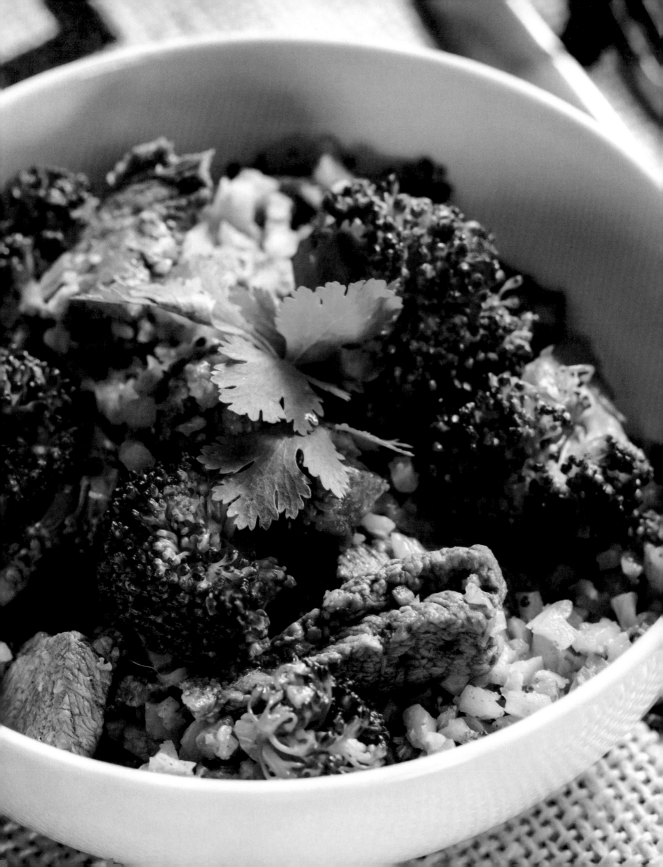

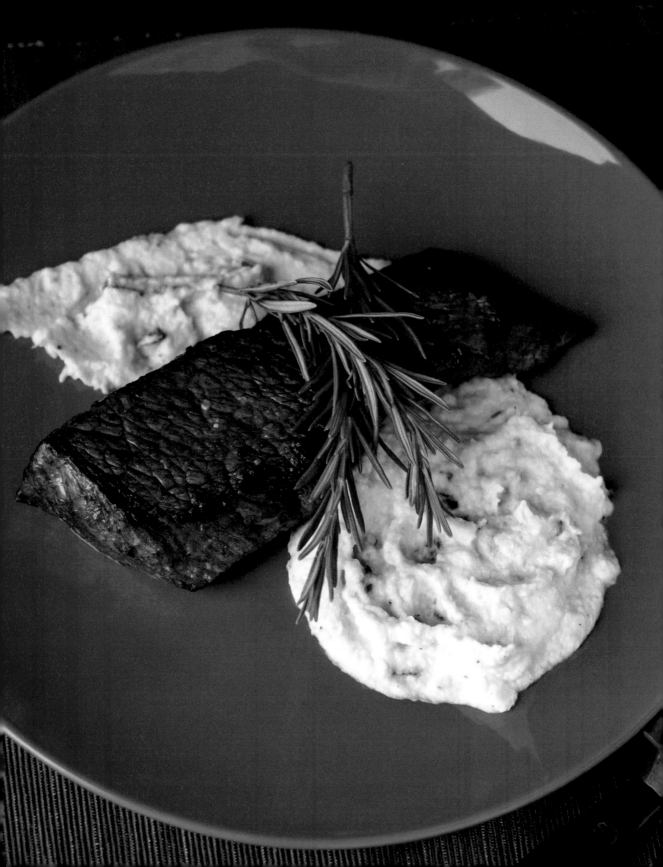

BEEF TOP ROUND STEAK
WITH GARLIC CAULIFLOWER MASH

MAKES 1 SERVING

658 calories | 49g fat | 11g carbs | 48g protein

6 ounces beef top round steak

Sea salt and pepper, to taste

1 tablespoon ghee

2 cups cauliflower

2 tablespoons unsweetened cashew milk (or dairy-free milk alternative)

1 tablespoon garlic-infused olive oil

½ teaspoon garlic powder

2 slices bacon, cooked and chopped

About a half hour prior to preparing dinner, set out the steak on a countertop and allow it to come to room temperature. This allows for more even cooking and tenderness.

When it is time to prepare, pat the steak with paper towel. Season on both sides with sea salt and pepper, using your hands to rub in.

Heat the ghee in a large skillet for about 1 minute over high heat. Add the steak and allow it to sear for 3 to 4 minutes for medium rare; flip and sear it for another 3 to 4 minutes. *(Cooking time depends on desired doneness.)*

Meanwhile, steam the cauliflower until it is soft. *(You can do this by cooking in the microwave with a few tablespoons of water for 5 to 6 minutes.)*

Once the cauliflower is soft, drain any excess water from the dish. Place the steamed cauliflower in a blender or food processor and add the remaining ingredients, except for the bacon.

Blend until smooth. Place the mash on a plate and sprinkle with bacon.

Enjoy the top round steak with cauliflower mash on the side.

BUFFALO WINGS & COLESLAW

MAKES 1 SERVING

660 calories | 53g fat | 10g carbs | 35g protein

6 ounces chicken wings

Garlic powder, to taste

Sea salt and pepper, to taste

¼ cup buffalo sauce

1 cup chopped broccoli

1 tablespoon avocado oil

FOR THE COLESLAW:

2 cups shredded cabbage

1½ tablespoons paleo mayo

1 teaspoon mustard

½ teaspoon apple cider vinegar

Pinch of stevia

Preheat the oven to 375 degrees Fahrenheit, line a baking sheet with foil for easy cleanup, and spray it with nonstick cooking spray. Set it aside.

Combine the chicken wings in a large bowl with garlic powder, sea salt, and pepper to taste, and toss until evenly seasoned. Add the buffalo sauce and toss again until the wings are well coated.

Lay the wings on a baking sheet, careful that no pieces overlap. Bake in the preheated oven for 1 hour, or until the wings are cooked through and have an internal temperature of 165 degrees Fahrenheit.

Meanwhile, as the wings are cooking, place the cabbage, mayo, mustard, vinegar, and stevia in a bowl. Mix until the cabbage is well coated. Season with sea salt and pepper to taste. Chill the coleslaw in the refrigerator until ready to serve.

Once the wings are cooked, set them aside and allow them to cool for 5 to 10 minutes. While they are cooling, add the broccoli and avocado oil to a skillet with additional garlic powder, sea salt, and pepper to taste. Sauté until the broccoli is bright green and just beginning to soften, about 5 to 8 minutes.

Serve the wings with the broccoli and coleslaw on the side, and enjoy!

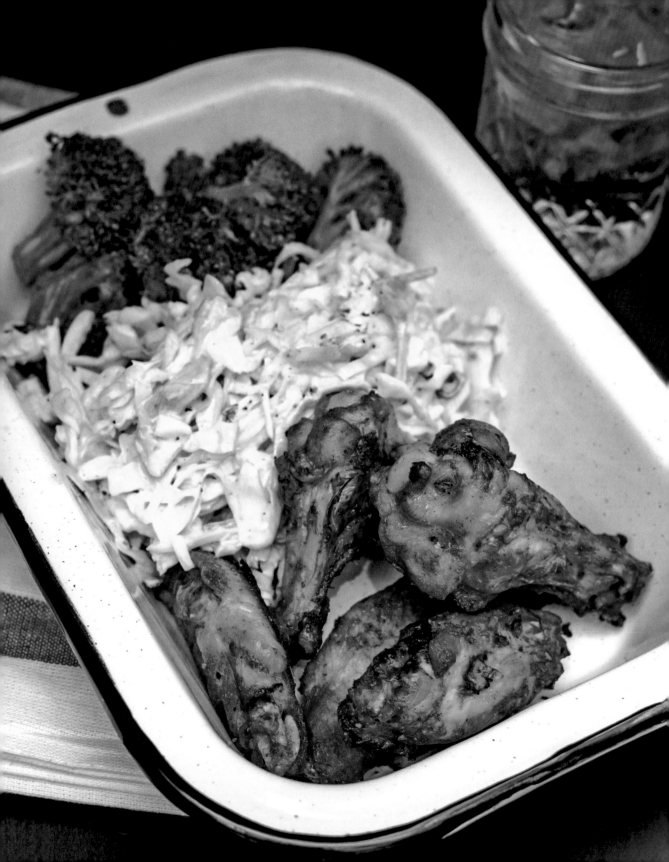

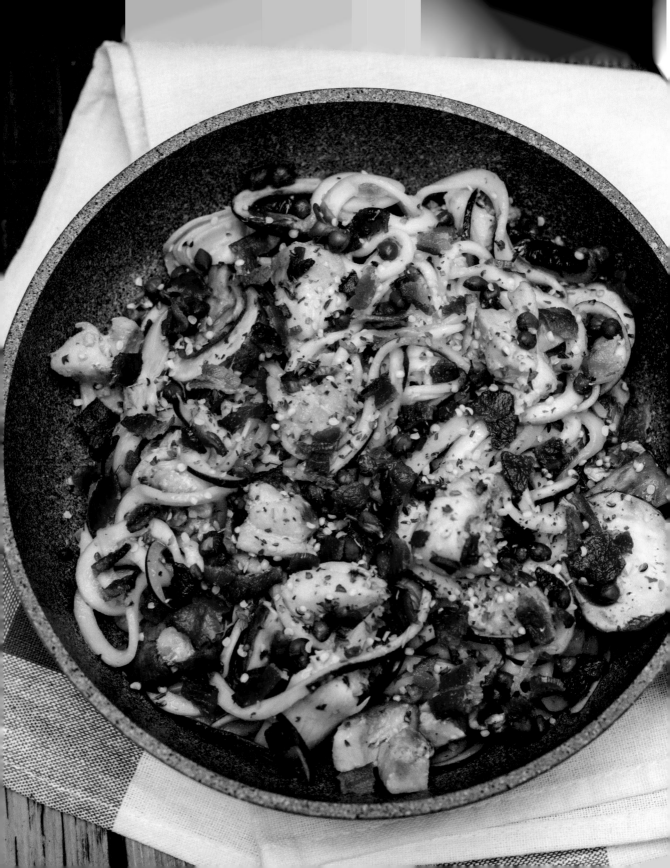

CHICKEN ARTICHOKE ZOODLE PAN

MAKES 1 SERVING

653 calories | 51g fat | 13g carbs | 37g protein

5 ounces boneless chicken thighs, chopped

2 slices bacon, chopped

2 tablespoons avocado oil

1 teaspoon minced garlic

Sea salt and pepper, to taste

½ cup baby bella mushrooms

¼ cup artichoke hearts

5 ounces zoodles

1 teaspoon Italian seasoning

Fresh thyme, to taste

Parsley, to taste

1 tablespoon hemp hearts

2 tablespoons capers

Mix the chicken thighs, bacon, 1 tablespoon of avocado oil, minced garlic, sea salt, and pepper in a skillet. Toss until well coated in seasonings and oil. Cook over medium heat until cooked through, about 7 to 9 minutes, or until chicken reaches an internal temperature of 165 degrees Fahrenheit. Set aside.

Meanwhile, add the remaining avocado oil, mushrooms, artichoke hearts, zoodles, and remaining seasonings to the skillet. Sauté until the mushrooms are soft and the zoodles are bright green.

Add the chicken and bacon mixture back to the skillet and toss until mixed well. Then remove it from the heat.

Sprinkle with hemp hearts and capers, and enjoy immediately!

CHIPOTLE PORTOBELLO MUSHROOM BURGER

MAKES 1 SERVING

614 calories | 50g fat | 11g carbs | 35g protein

⅓-pound (5.3-ounce) ground sirloin hamburger patty

Sea salt and pepper, to taste

Garlic and herb seasoning, to taste

Two 4-ounce portobello mushroom caps

½ tablespoon olive oil

Smoked paprika, to taste

1 cup chopped broccoli

½ tablespoon ghee

1 tablespoon paleo mayo

½ teaspoon Dijon mustard

½ teaspoon chipotle seasoning

1 to 2 lettuce leaves

Preheat grill to medium heat.

As your grill is heating, season the hamburger patty with sea salt, pepper, and garlic and herb seasoning on both sides.

Rub the mushroom caps with olive oil on both sides, then season them with sea salt, pepper, and smoked paprika.

Grill the hamburger and mushroom caps on the preheated grill, and cook until they have the desired doneness and texture.

Meanwhile, sauté the broccoli in ghee in a skillet over medium heat. Season with sea salt and pepper, and continue tossing until broccoli is just soft and bright green, about 5 to 7 minutes.

Combine the paleo mayo, mustard, and chipotle seasoning in a small bowl. Mix until well combined. Chill in refrigerator until ready to serve.

Once the hamburger is cooked to desired doneness, place it on top of a grilled portobello mushroom cap, and top with chipotle mayo and lettuce and the second mushroom cap. Enjoy it with broccoli on the side!

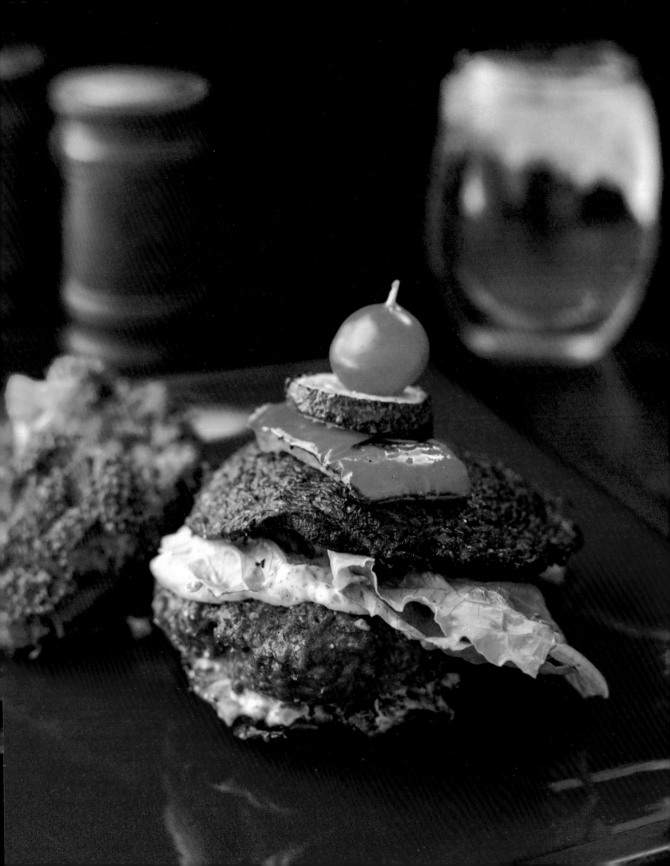

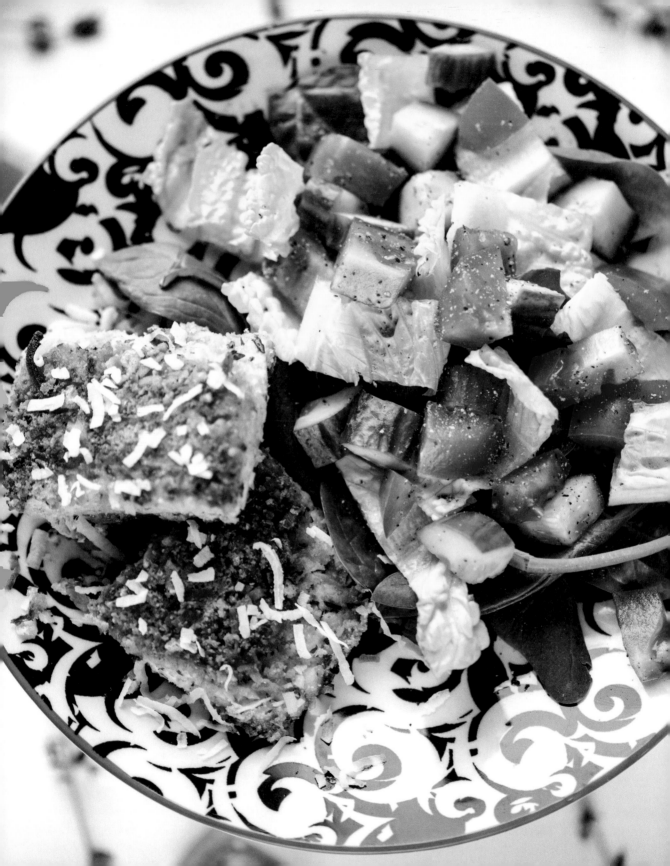

COCONUT-CRUSTED SALMON
WITH SPRING SALAD

737 calories | 60g fat | 12g carbs | 41g protein

1 tablespoon coconut flour

1 tablespoon unsweetened shredded coconut

1 teaspoon dried parsley

½ ounce pork rinds, crushed fine

½ teaspoon stevia

¼ teaspoon garlic powder

Sea salt and pepper, to taste

1½ tablespoons coconut oil

6-ounce wild-caught salmon fillet

2 cups chopped hearts of romaine and spinach

¼ cup diced cucumbers

¼ cup diced tomatoes

½ tablespoon avocado oil

Apple cider vinegar, to taste

In a small, wide bowl, combine the coconut flour, coconut, parsley, crushed pork rinds, stevia, garlic powder, sea salt, and pepper. Mix until they are well combined.

Over medium-high heat, melt the coconut oil, and allow it to heat a minute or two.

Meanwhile, dip the salmon in the coconut flour mixture, coating both sides well.

Place the salmon in heated coconut oil, skin side down. Allow it to cook about 5 minutes, and then flip it. Continue frying it for another 5 to 6 minutes or until it reaches an internal temperature of 145 degrees Fahrenheit.

Remove the salmon from the oil and transfer to a plate.

Place the greens, cucumbers, tomatoes, avocado oil, and apple cider vinegar in a bowl. Toss until well combined.

Enjoy the salmon with salad on the side.

CREAMY SALMON FILLET

MAKES 1 SERVING

635 calories | 53g fat | 7g carbs | 35g protein

7-ounce wild-caught salmon fillet

1 tablespoon paleo mayo

Blend of your favorite fresh herbs, chopped

Sea salt and pepper, to taste

1 cup asparagus

1 tablespoon avocado oil

Preheat the oven to 375 degrees Fahrenheit, line a baking sheet with foil, and spray it with nonstick cooking spray.

Place the salmon fillet on the baking sheet, spread the mayo on top, and sprinkle with the chopped herbs and sea salt and pepper to taste. Bake in the preheated oven for 15 to 20 minutes, until the salmon is cooked through and flaking or reaches an internal temperature of 145 degrees Fahrenheit.

While the salmon is cooking, sauté the asparagus in avocado oil over medium heat and season to taste with salt and pepper.

Enjoy the salmon with asparagus on the side!

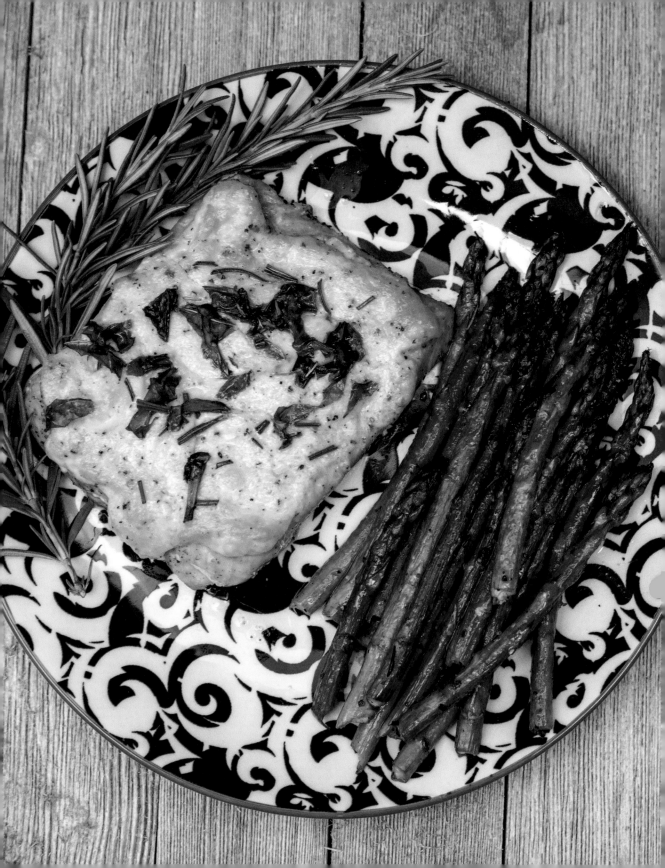

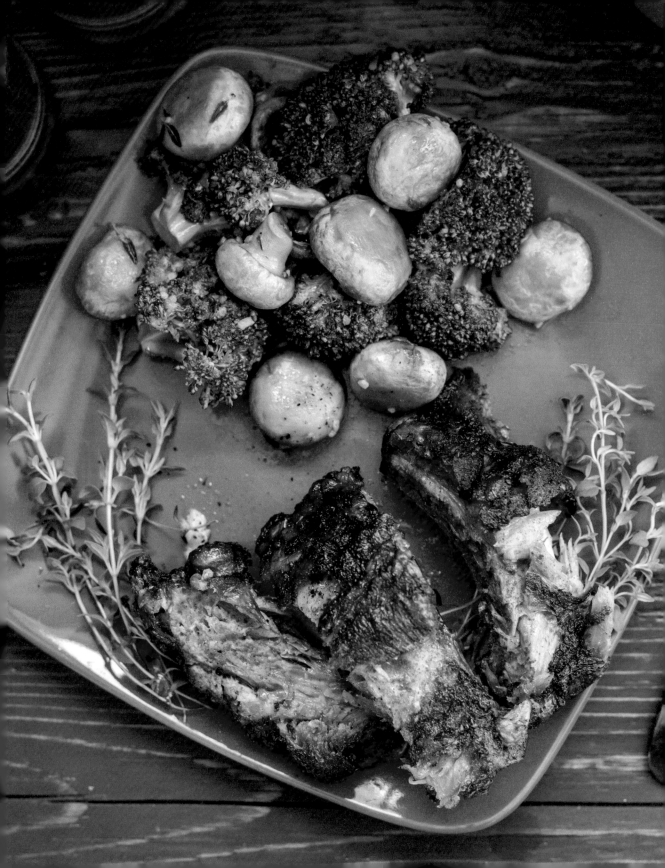

DRY RUB RIBS
& LEMON GARLIC ROASTED VEGETABLES

699 calories | 60g fat | 11g carbs | 32g protein

5 ounces baby back pork ribs

2 tablespoons avocado oil

1 cup button mushrooms

1 cup chopped broccoli

Sea salt and pepper, to taste

1 teaspoon fresh thyme, chopped

½ teaspoon minced garlic

½ tablespoon lemon juice

FOR THE RIB RUB:

½ tablespoon instant coffee grounds

½ teaspoon sea salt

¼ teaspoon black pepper

½ teaspoon garlic powder

½ teaspoon onion powder

¼ teaspoon oregano

Pinch of paprika

Pinch of cayenne (optional)

Stevia, to taste

Preheat oven to 250 degrees Fahrenheit. Line a baking dish with foil and set aside.

Pat the ribs dry with a paper towel and rub 1 tablespoon of the avocado oil on both sides.

In a small dish, combine all the ingredients for the rub together. Season the ribs on both sides to taste with the rub.

Place the ribs on the foil-lined baking dish and wrap them tightly in the foil, securely covering the ribs. Place them on a baking sheet and cook in the preheated oven for 2½ hours.

While the ribs are cooking, place the vegetables in a large bowl. Season with sea salt, pepper, thyme, and garlic, and drizzle with remaining 1 tablespoon of avocado oil and lemon juice. Toss until the vegetables are evenly coated, and place them on a baking sheet, being careful that none overlap. Set aside.

Remove the ribs from the oven and open the foil; be careful to not burn yourself, as steam will release. Turn the oven up to 350 degrees Fahrenheit.

Remove the ribs from the foil, place them on the baking sheet, and return them to the oven for another ½ hour.

Place the vegetables in the oven with ribs, and allow to cook the remaining ½ hour.

Allow the ribs to cool 5 to 10 minutes. Enjoy with roasted vegetables on the side.

FILET MIGNON
WITH ROASTED CAULIFLOWER

MAKES 1 SERVING

686 calories | 55g fat | 8g carbs | 40g protein

5-ounce filet mignon steak

Sea salt and pepper, to taste

Cumin, to taste

Smoked paprika, to taste

Garlic powder, to taste

1½ cups cauliflower

2 tablespoons ghee

Preheat grill. Season the steak with the suggested seasonings on each side, using your fingers to rub them in.

Grill over medium heat to desired doneness.

Meanwhile, preheat the oven to 450 degrees Fahrenheit. Toss the cauliflower in 1 tablespoon of melted ghee, and season with sea salt and pepper. Lay the cauliflower on a baking sheet and roast for 10 to 15 minutes, or until soft and browning around the edges.

Serve the steak topped with the remaining ghee and the cauliflower on the side.

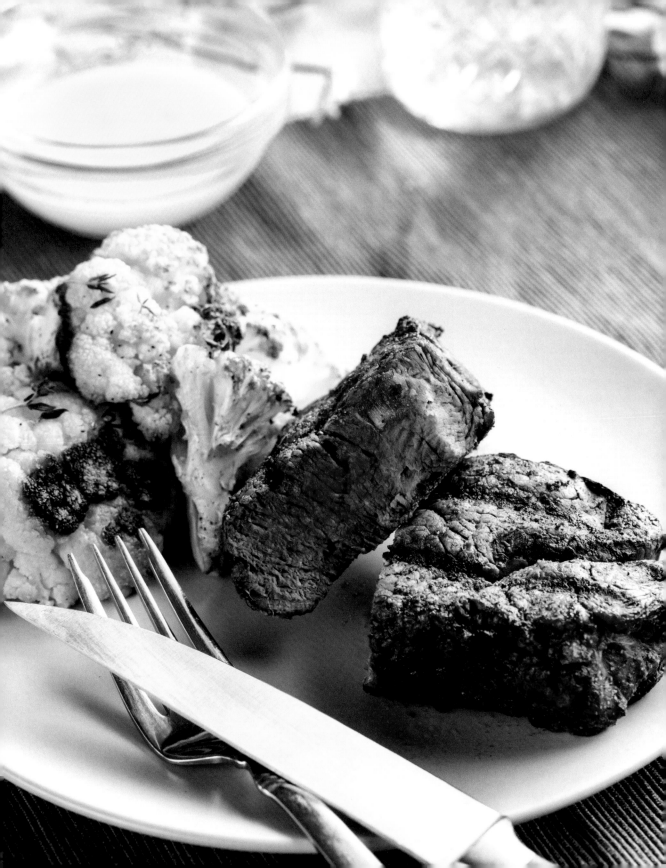

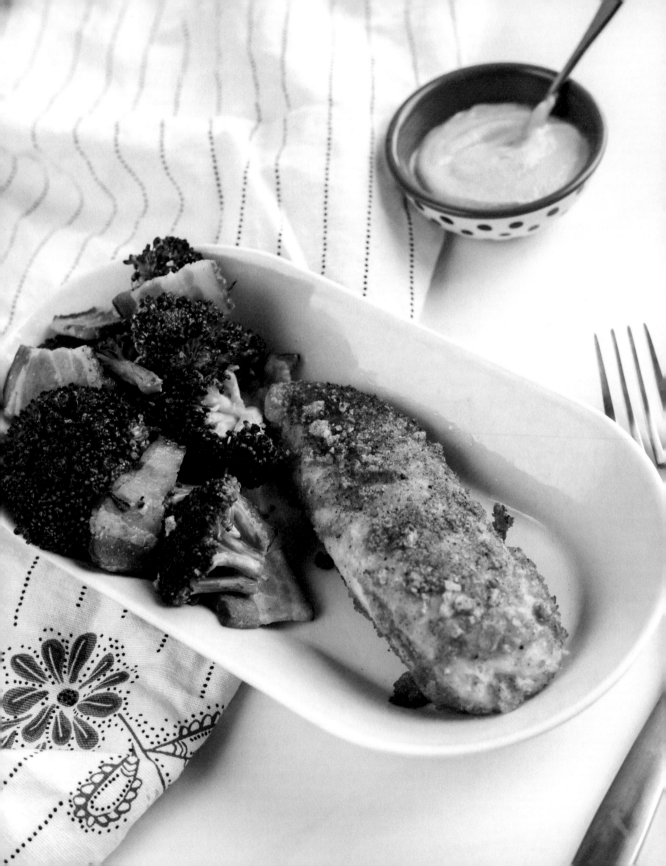

FRIED CHICKEN & BACON BROCCOLI

MAKES 1 SERVING

707 calories | 48g fat | 14g carbs | 39g protein

2 tablespoons coconut flour

1 ounce pork rinds, crushed fine

Smoked paprika, to taste

Sea salt and pepper, to taste

1 egg

4-ounce chicken breast

¼ cup + ½ tablespoon avocado oil

1 cup broccoli

2 slices bacon, chopped

Combine 1 tablespoon of coconut flour, crushed pork rinds, and seasonings in a bowl. Mix well. Beat 1 egg in a separate bowl and set it aside.

Dip the chicken in the remaining flour, coating both sides well. Then dip it into the egg, careful to coat both sides. Then dip the chicken into the pork rind mixture, coating both sides until well covered.

Heat ¼ cup avocado oil in a skillet over medium-high heat. Add the chicken breast to the oil and allow it to fry for about 4 to 5 minutes on one side before flipping. Allow it to cook another 3 to 4 minutes, or until the chicken is cooked through and reaches an internal temperature of 165 degrees Fahrenheit.

Meanwhile, add the remaining avocado oil to a skillet. Add the broccoli and bacon, and season with sea salt to taste. Toss until well coated, and cook until the broccoli is bright green and the bacon is cooked through, about 5 to 6 minutes.

Serve the fried chicken with bacon and broccoli on the side, and enjoy!

GARLIC & HERB FLANK STEAK
WITH BROCCOLI

MAKES 1 SERVING

605 calories | 40g fat | 6g carbs | 52g protein

8-ounce flank steak

Garlic powder, to taste

Paprika, to taste

Cumin, to taste

Sea salt and pepper, to taste

1 tablespoon ghee

¼ teaspoon minced garlic

1 teaspoon of your favorite fresh herbs, minced

1½ cups broccoli

½ tablespoon olive oil

Preheat grill to medium heat. While it is heating, season the steak on each side with garlic powder, paprika, cumin, sea salt, and pepper, to taste.

Grill on the preheated grill to desired doneness.

Meanwhile, in a small bowl, combine the ghee, minced garlic, and minced herbs. Mix until thoroughly combined, and set aside.

In a skillet, sauté the broccoli in the olive oil and season with sea salt and pepper. Cook until the broccoli is bright green and just soft.

Once the steak is cooked to desired doneness, top it with the ghee-and-garlic blend and serve with broccoli on the side. Enjoy!

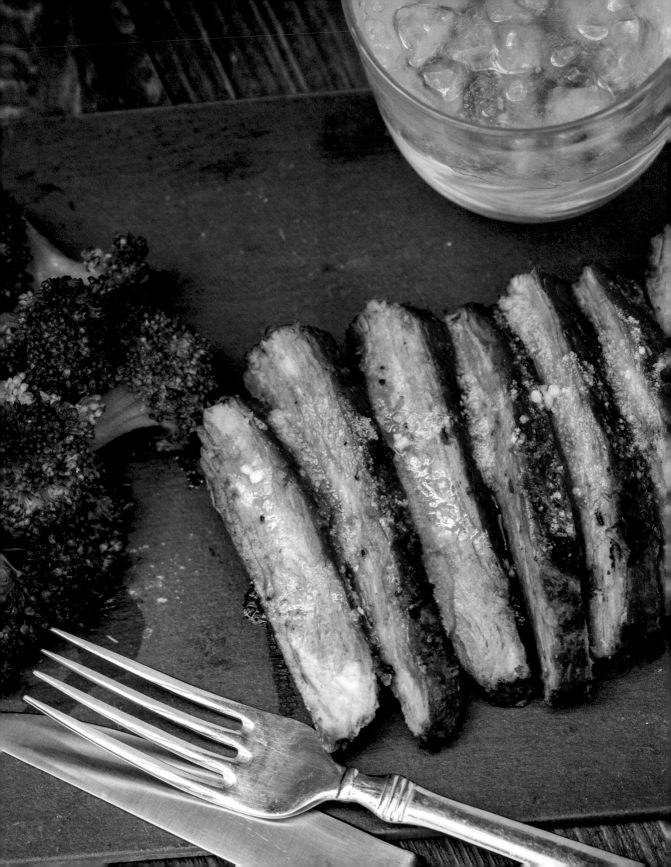

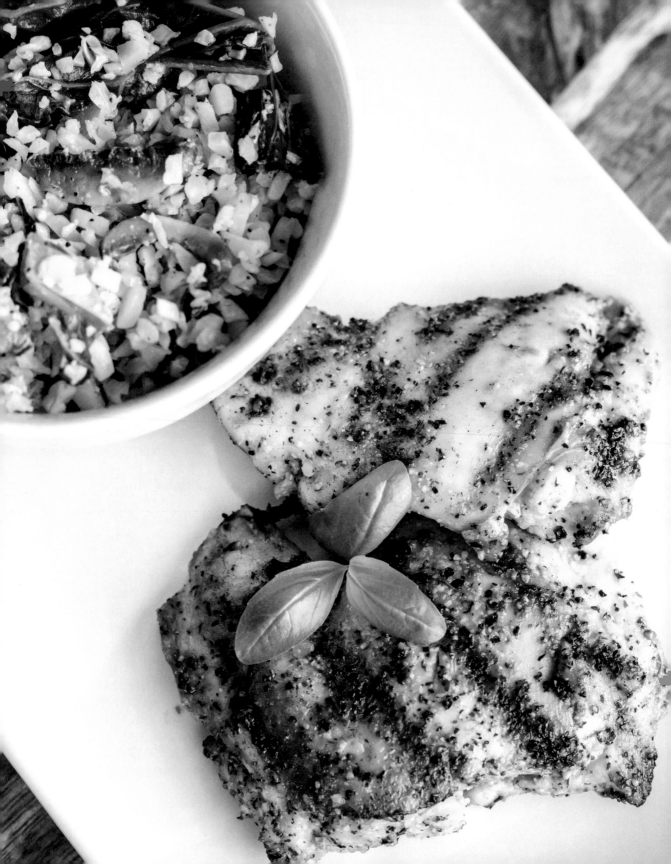

GRILLED CHICKEN THIGHS
WITH SAUTÉED CAULIFLOWER MEDLEY

MAKES 1 SERVING

515 calories | 36g fat | 9g carbs | 37g protein

6 ounces boneless, skinless chicken thighs

1 tablespoon avocado oil

Sea salt and pepper, to taste

Garlic and herb seasoning blend, to taste

1 tablespoon ghee

½ teaspoon minced garlic

1 cup collard greens

1 cup cauliflower rice

⅓ cup sliced mushrooms

Lay the chicken thighs on a baking sheet and pat them dry with a paper towel. Using your fingers, rub the chicken with avocado oil on each side. Season with sea salt, pepper, and garlic and herb seasoning on each side, to taste.

Preheat the grill to medium heat (or you may also cook in an oven if preferred). Grill the chicken thighs until they reach an internal temperature of 165 degrees Fahrenheit, about 25 minutes. Be sure to flip them once halfway through cooking. Remove them from the heat and cover them until ready to serve.

Meanwhile, melt the ghee in a skillet over medium heat. Add the minced garlic and sauté briefly until fragrant, about 2 to 3 minutes. Add in the collard greens, cauliflower rice, and mushrooms. Season with sea salt and pepper, and continue to sauté until the cauliflower is just beginning to discolor and the collard greens are wilted, about 5 to 8 minutes.

Serve with the chicken thighs on a plate and enjoy!

GRILLED RIB EYE & ASPARAGUS

MAKES 1 SERVING

597 calories | 47g fat | 10g carbs | 37g protein

6-ounce rib eye steak

Paprika, to taste

Cumin, to taste

Garlic powder, to taste

Sea salt and pepper, to taste

2 cups asparagus

1 tablespoon avocado oil

1 tablespoon ghee

Preheat grill. Season the steak with the suggested seasonings on each side, using your fingers to rub them in.

Grill over medium heat to desired doneness.

Meanwhile, sauté the asparagus in avocado oil over medium-low heat, and season to taste with salt and pepper. Continue cooking until the asparagus is just soft and bright green, about 7 to 9 minutes.

Top the steak with the ghee and serve with the asparagus on the side. Enjoy!

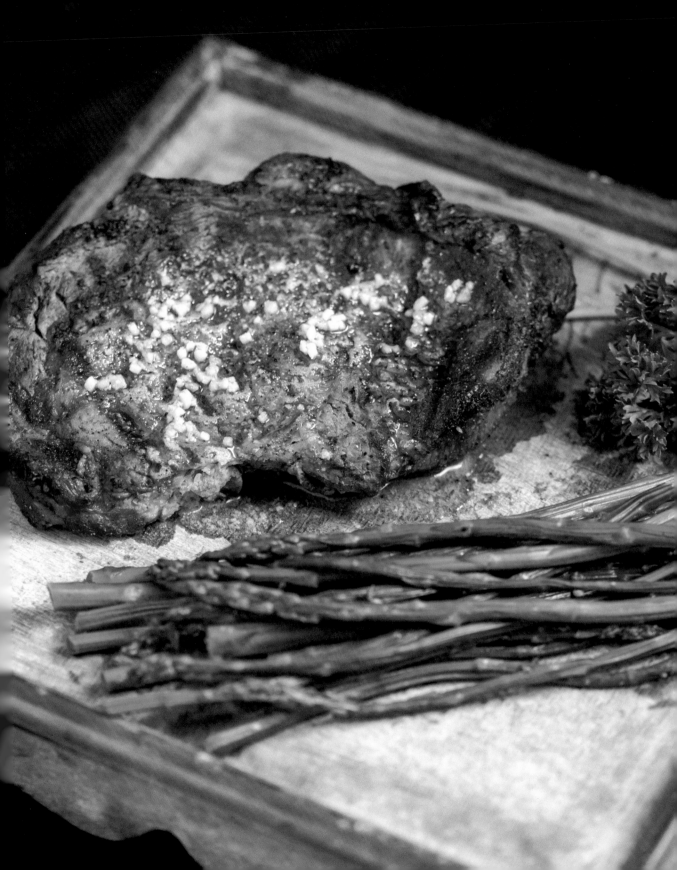

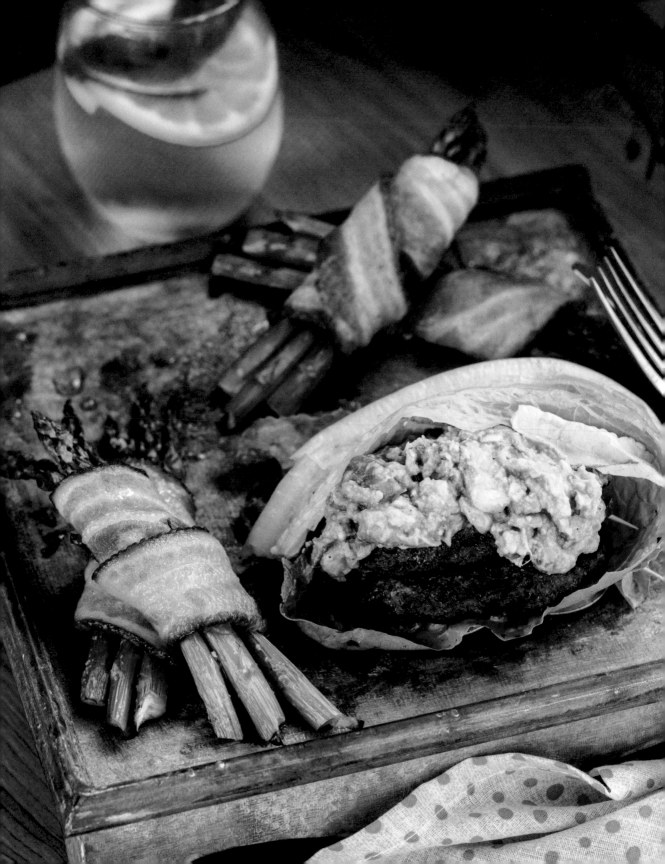

GUACAMOLE BURGER
with BACON-WRAPPED ASPARAGUS STACKS

MAKES 1 SERVING

644 calories | 50g fat | 14g carbs | 36g protein

4 ounces grass-fed ground beef

Sea salt and pepper, to taste

Cumin, to taste

Paprika, to taste

1½ cups asparagus

1 tablespoon avocado oil

3 slices bacon

1 lettuce leaf

¼ cup guacamole

Preheat grill and season ground beef with seasonings. Form beef into a patty to desired thickness and grill over medium-high heat for 4 to 5 minutes on one side. Then flip and continue cooking for another 4 minutes, or to desired doneness.

Meanwhile, preheat oven to 400 degrees Fahrenheit and line a baking sheet with parchment paper or foil. Toss the asparagus with avocado oil, sea salt, and pepper. Divide the asparagus into 3 stacks, and wrap each stack with bacon. Place the asparagus on the baking sheet and bake in preheated oven for 20 to 25 minutes.

Wrap the hamburger with lettuce and top with guacamole. Enjoy with the asparagus stacks on the side.

JAMBALAYA

MAKES 1 SERVING

649 calories | 50g fat | 19g carbs | 31g protein

2 ounces boneless, skinless chicken thighs, chopped

Sea salt and pepper, to taste

1 tablespoon ghee

1 chicken andouille sausage, chopped

1 tablespoon avocado oil

¼ cup diced bell pepper

¼ cup diced onion

½ cup diced celery

½ cup low-carb marinara sauce

¼ teaspoon paprika

¼ teaspoon Cajun seasoning

¼ teaspoon dried oregano

¼ teaspoon dried thyme

Red pepper flakes, to taste (optional)

1½ cups cauliflower rice

Season the chicken with sea salt and pepper, to taste. Melt ½ tablespoon of ghee in a large skillet over medium heat. Add the chicken and cook until it's no longer pink in the center, about 5 to 8 minutes. Set it aside.

Melt the remaining ghee and fry the chicken sausage until its edges are just browned, and then set it aside.

Add ½ tablespoon avocado oil to the same pan, then add the pepper, onion, and celery. Sauté for about 5 minutes until vegetables are just soft. Add the low-carb marinara sauce and seasonings. Add the sausage and chicken back into the pan. Turn the heat down to low, and allow to simmer for about 3 minutes.

Meanwhile, add the remaining oil and cauliflower rice to a small skillet over medium heat. Sauté the cauliflower until it just begins to color, about 5 minutes. Remove from heat and place in a bowl.

Top the cauliflower rice with the jambalaya and enjoy!

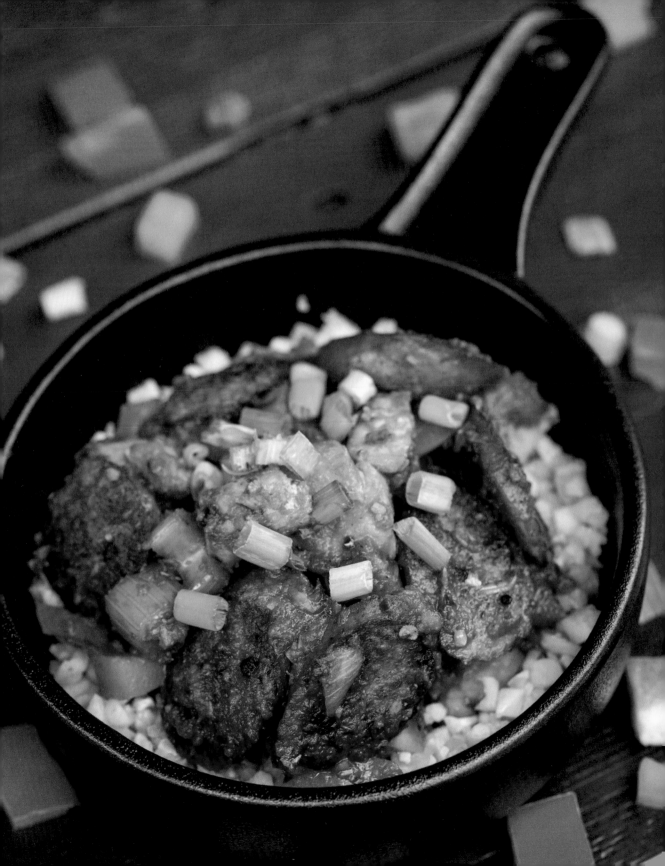

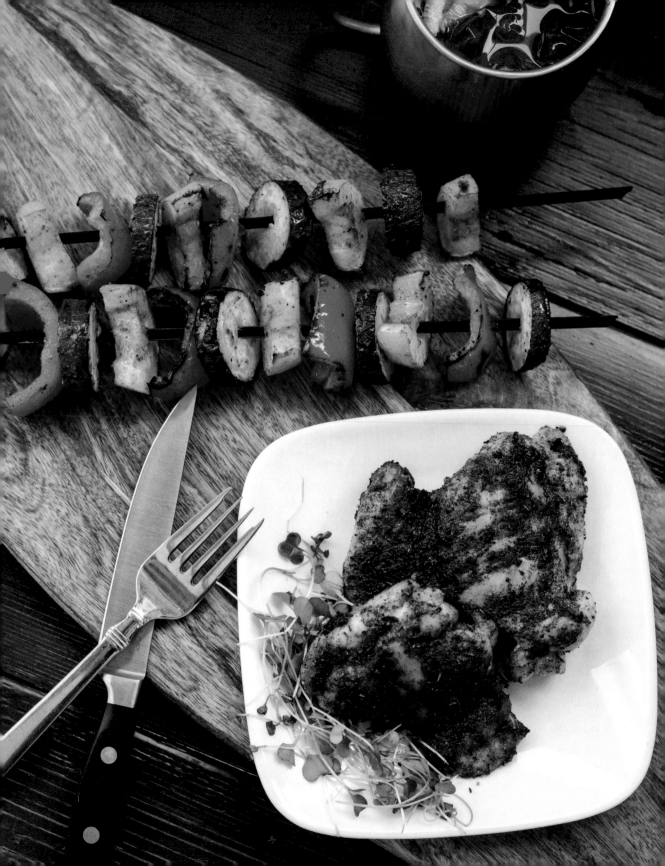

JERK CHICKEN & VEGGIE KABOBS

MAKES 1 SERVING

650 calories | 53g fat | 10g carbs | 32g protein

4 ounces bone-in chicken thighs

2 tablespoons olive oil

½ medium zucchini, sliced

½ medium yellow squash, sliced

½ medium red bell pepper, sliced

¼ teaspoon garlic powder

¼ teaspoon paprika

Sea salt and pepper, to taste

FOR SEASONING BLEND:

2 teaspoons allspice

½ teaspoon nutmeg

1 teaspoon sea salt

½ teaspoon stevia

2 teaspoons dried thyme

1 teaspoon ground ginger

1 teaspoon pepper

1 teaspoon garlic powder

1 teaspoon onion powder

¼ teaspoon red pepper flakes (optional)

Preheat grill to medium-high heat.

Meanwhile, combine all the spices for the seasoning blend in a small bowl and mix well. Set aside.

Pat the chicken thighs dry with a paper towel, then baste them with 1 tablespoon of olive oil on each side. Season with the seasoning blend to taste. (I recommend 1 to 2 teaspoons.) Allow chicken to rest about 15 minutes.

Place the vegetables in a large bowl and drizzle with the remaining olive oil. Season with the remaining seasonings and toss until well coated. Place the vegetables on skewers for grilling and set aside.

Place the chicken thighs skin side down on grill. Allow them to cook for 5 to 6 minutes, and then flip them. Grill them for about 5 minutes, and then flip them again. Continue this pattern for about 25 to 30 minutes or until the chicken thighs reach an internal temperature of 165 degrees Fahrenheit.

About 10 to 15 minutes into grilling the chicken, add the vegetable skewers to the grill, flipping it at the same time as the chicken. Remove it from the heat once its edges begin to blacken and the vegetables are soft. Depending on the grill, this may be sooner than when the chicken is done. Keep a close eye and remove when desired.

Allow the chicken to rest about 5 to 10 minutes after removing it from the grill, and enjoy it with the veggie kabob on the side!

KETO CHICKEN CHOW MEIN

MAKES 1 SERVING

657 calories | 51g fat | 13g carbs | 36g protein

1½ tablespoons avocado oil

1 teaspoon minced garlic

4 ounces boneless, skinless chicken thighs, chopped

Sea salt and pepper, to taste

2 ounces ground pork sausage, cooked

5 ounces zoodles

1 cup shredded cabbage

⅓ cup sliced mushrooms

¼ cup chopped green onion

2 teaspoons coconut aminos

2 teaspoons sesame oil

1 teaspoon white wine vinegar

¼ teaspoon ground ginger

Heat ½ tablespoon of avocado oil in a large frying pan, add the minced garlic, and sauté until fragrant. Add the chicken, sea salt, and pepper, and continue cooking until chicken is cooked through or reaches an internal temperature of 165 degrees Fahrenheit. Remove from the pan and set aside.

Add the remaining avocado oil and the rest of the ingredients to the frying pan. Toss until everything is well combined. Cook for about 5 to 7 minutes, or until the cabbage is wilted and the zoodles are bright green.

Remove from the heat and add the chicken, mixing until well combined. Enjoy!

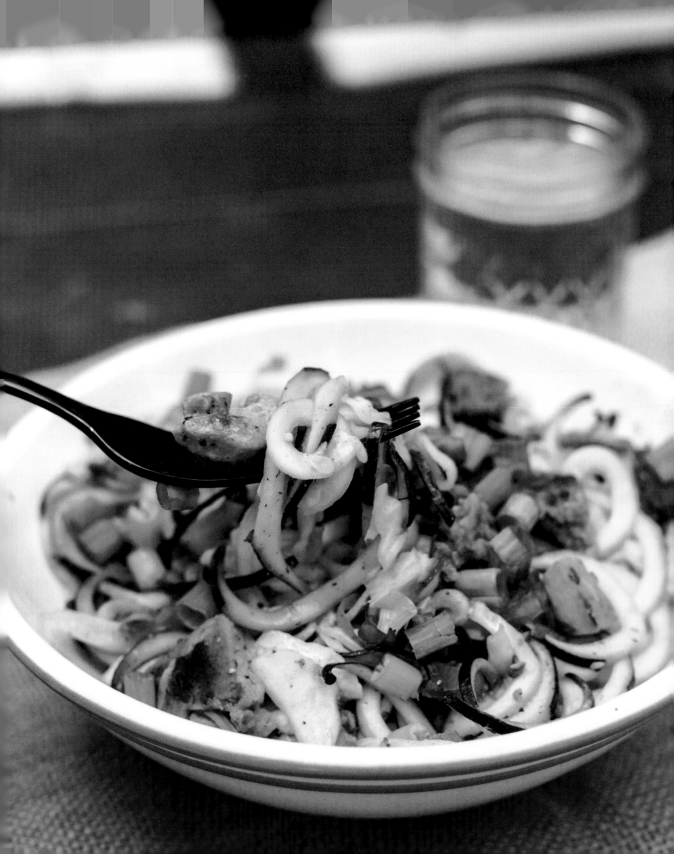

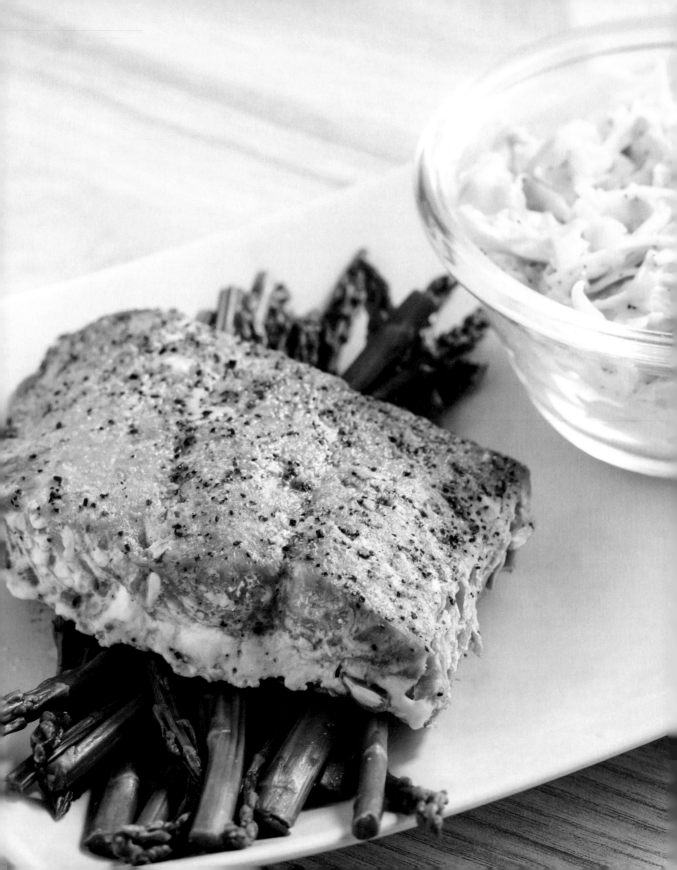

LEMON PEPPER SALMON
with COLESLAW & ASPARAGUS

MAKES 1 SERVING

722 calories | 63g fat | 12g carbs | 32g protein

6 ounces wild-caught salmon

2 tablespoons avocado oil

Sea salt and pepper, to taste

Lemon pepper, to taste

1 teaspoon lemon juice

1 cup shredded cabbage

1 tablespoon paleo mayo

1 teaspoon mustard

1 teaspoon apple cider vinegar

Pinch of stevia

1 cup steamed asparagus

Preheat the oven to 400 degrees Fahrenheit.

Rub the salmon on both sides with 1 tablespoon of avocado oil, and season to taste with sea salt and lemon pepper. Place on a greased baking sheet, skin side down, and sprinkle with lemon juice. Bake in the preheated oven for 12 to 15 minutes, until the salmon is flaky and reaches an internal temperature of 145 degrees Fahrenheit.

Meanwhile, as the salmon is cooking, place the cabbage, mayo, mustard, vinegar, and stevia in a bowl. Toss until well coated, and season with sea salt and pepper to taste. Chill in the refrigerator until it's ready to serve.

Toss the steamed asparagus in the remaining 1 tablespoon avocado oil, and season with sea salt.

Serve the salmon with the asparagus and coleslaw on the side.

POLISH SAUSAGE
WITH FRIED CABBAGE & COLLARD GREENS

MAKES 1 SERVING

561 calories | 43g fat | 11g carbs | 33g protein

1½ tablespoons avocado oil

1 teaspoon chopped garlic

2 Polish sausage links (128 grams or 4½ ounces), cut into bite-size pieces

2 cups shredded cabbage

2 cups collard greens

1 tablespoon red wine vinegar

Sea salt and pepper, to taste

Paprika, to taste

Red pepper flakes, to taste (optional)

Put ½ tablespoon of avocado oil and garlic in a large skillet over medium heat. Sauté it until fragrant.

Add the Polish sausage and sauté until lightly browned around the edges.

Add the cabbage, collard greens, red wine vinegar, remaining oil, and seasonings. Toss until well coated with seasonings. Continue stirring and tossing until the cabbage and collard greens begin to wilt and brown slightly.

Remove it from the heat and allow it to cool a few minutes. Place it in a bowl and enjoy!

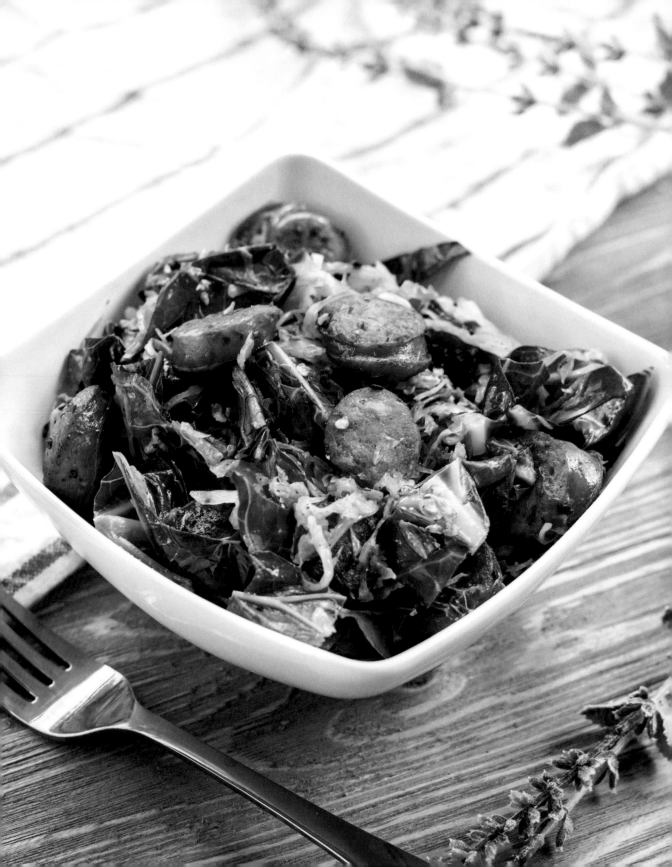

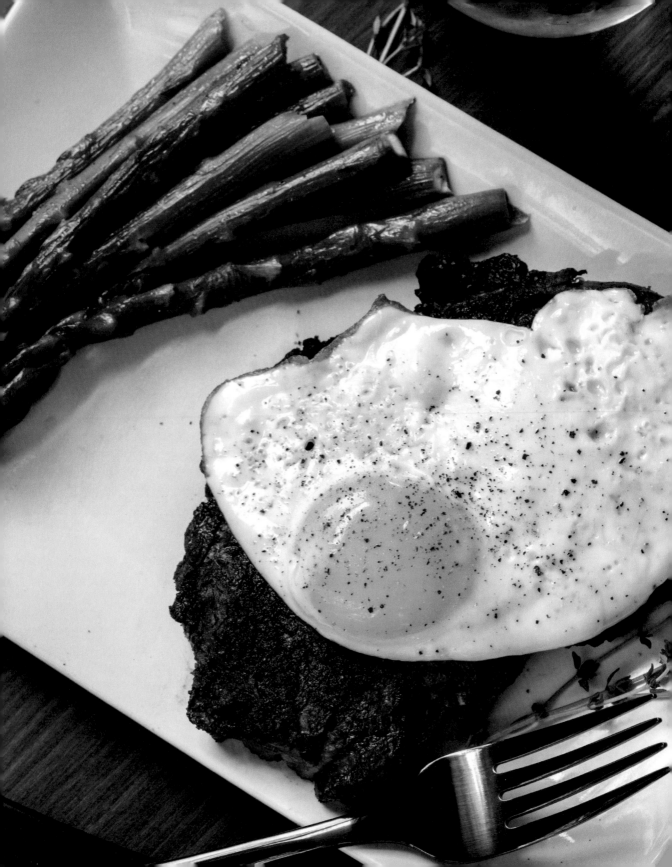

RIB EYE STEAK & EGG
WITH ASPARAGUS

MAKES 1 SERVING

532 calories | 38g fat | 8g carbs | 42g protein

6-ounce rib eye steak

Paprika, to taste

Cumin, to taste

Garlic powder, to taste

Sea salt and pepper, to taste

1½ cups asparagus

1 tablespoon ghee

1 egg

Preheat grill. Season the steak with the suggested seasonings on each side, using your fingers to rub them in.

Grill over medium heat to desired doneness.

Meanwhile, sauté the asparagus in ½ tablespoon of the ghee. Cook it over medium heat until it is bright green and just tender, about 5 to 8 minutes.

Melt the remaining ghee in a skillet over medium heat, and fry the egg to desired doneness.

Serve the steak topped with egg, with the asparagus on the side.

SMOKED CHILI PORK CHOP
WITH GREEN BEANS

MAKES 1 SERVING

557 calories | 39g fat | 9g carbs | 42g protein

¼ teaspoon sea salt

¼ teaspoon chili powder

¼ teaspoon smoked paprika

¼ teaspoon garlic powder

¼ teaspoon onion powder

Fresh cracked pepper, to taste

½ tablespoon olive oil

5-oz. bone-in pork loin chop

1 tablespoon ghee

1 cup fresh green beans

Preheat grill to medium heat.

Combine all the seasonings in a small bowl, and mix well.

Pour the olive oil on each side of the pork loin chop, using your fingers to rub it in until the pork chop is well coated.

Sprinkle the seasoning mixture on each side of the pork loin chop, and rub it in with your fingers, including the edges.

Grill on the preheated grill for 5 to 6 minutes on each side or until the pork reaches an internal temperature of 160 to 170 degrees Fahrenheit (160 for medium, 170 for well done).

Meanwhile, melt ghee over medium heat. Add green beans and season with sea salt and pepper. Sauté over medium heat until green beans are just soft, about 5–7 minutes.

Enjoy the pork chop with green beans on the side.

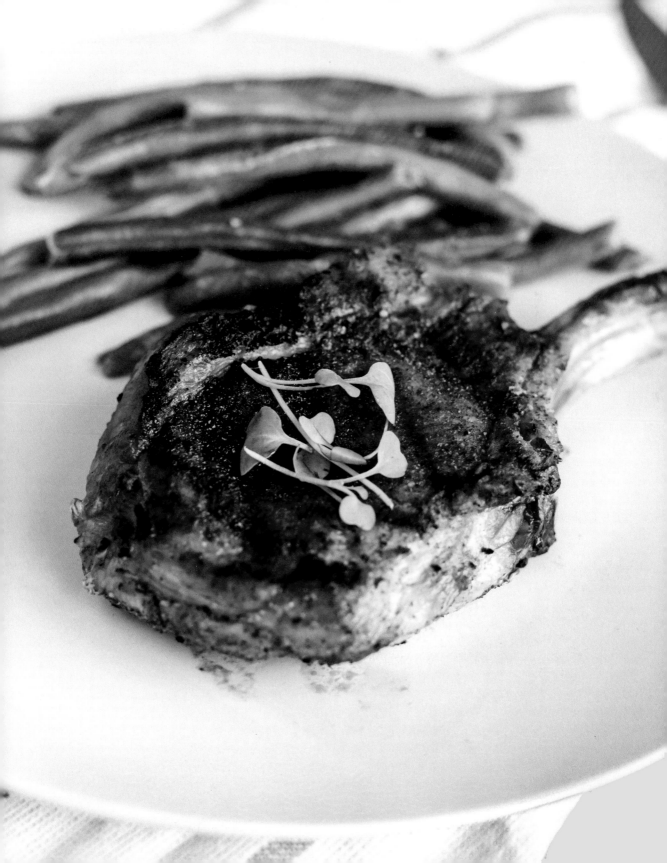

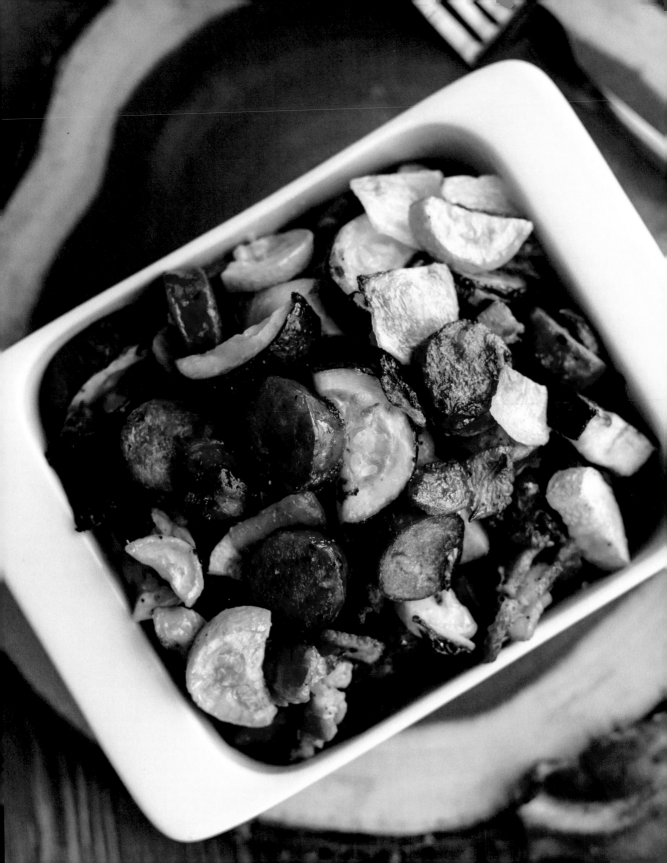

SMOKED SAUSAGE & ROASTED VEGETABLES

MAKES 1 SERVING

761 calories | 68g fat | 14g carbs | 28g protein

2 slices bacon, diced

1 cup chopped zucchini

½ cup chopped yellow squash

¼ cup chopped onion

2 tablespoons avocado oil

½ teaspoon garlic powder

1 teaspoon paprika

Sea salt and pepper, to taste

5 ounces andouille smoked sausage, sliced

Preheat oven to 425 degrees Fahrenheit, line a baking sheet with parchment paper, and set aside.

Combine all the ingredients in a large bowl and toss until well coated in the oil and seasonings.

Pour the sausage mixture on the baking sheet and spread evenly, being careful that the pieces do not overlap.

Bake in the preheated oven for 20 to 25 minutes, until the bacon is cooked through and the vegetables are soft.

Allow it to cool and enjoy!

UNSTUFFED PEPPERS

MAKES 1 SERVING

609 calories | 48g fat | 13g carbs | 30g protein

3 ounces ground beef chuck

2 ounces ground pork sausage

¼ teaspoon cumin

1 teaspoon minced garlic

1 tablespoon avocado oil

½ cup chopped bell pepper

½ cup sliced mushrooms

1 teaspoon Italian seasoning

Sea salt and pepper, to taste

1½ cups cauliflower rice

Put the ground beef chuck, sausage, cumin, and garlic in a large skillet over medium heat. Sauté until the ground beef is cooked through and no longer pink. Remove it from skillet and set it aside.

Add ½ tablespoon of avocado oil to the skillet, and swirl it around the bottom until well coated. Add the bell pepper, mushrooms, and remaining seasonings. Sauté until they are just soft.

Add the remaining avocado oil and cauliflower rice. Toss with the pepper mixture until well combined. Continue stirring and tossing until the cauliflower is slightly colored, and then remove from heat.

Add the meat and mix well. Allow to cool a few minutes; then place in a bowl and enjoy!

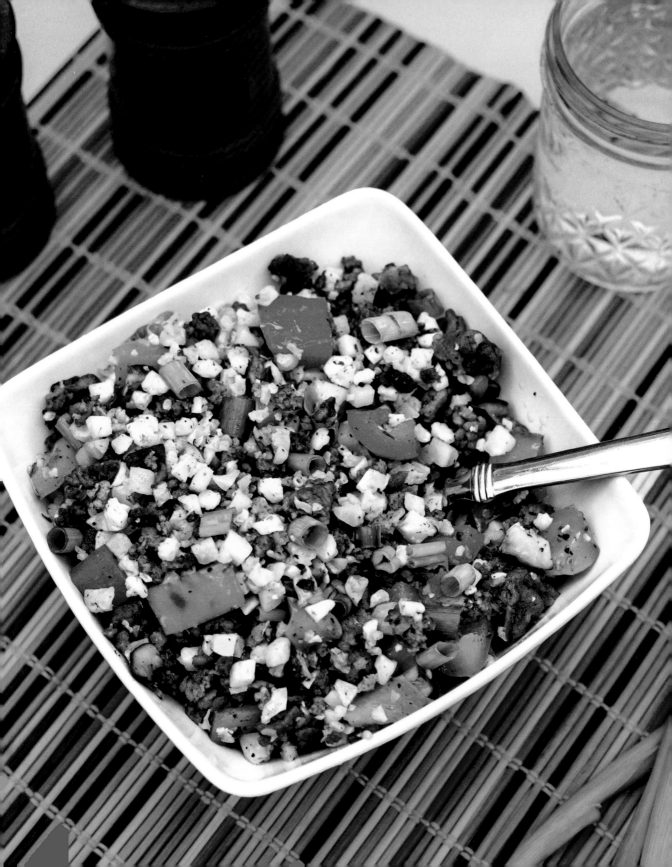

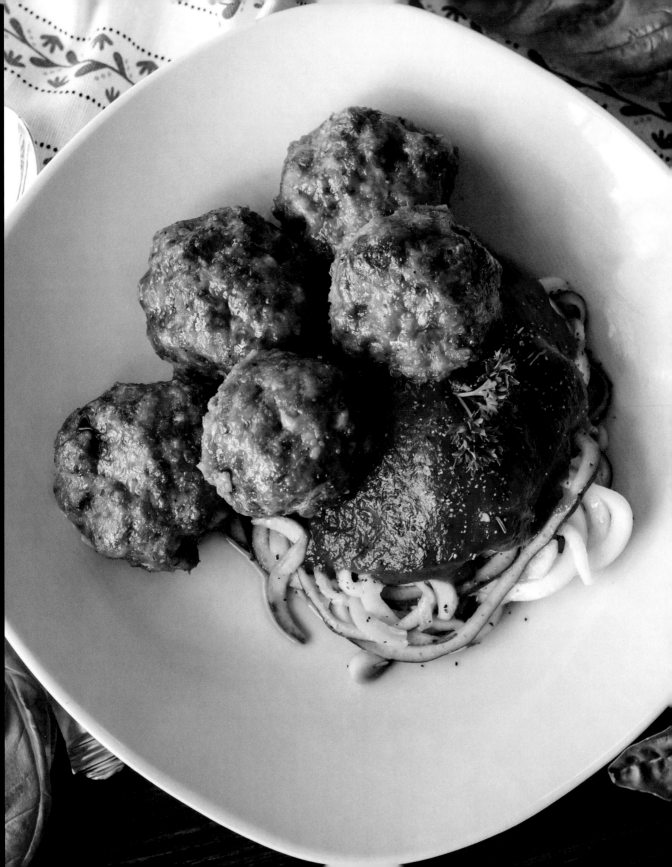

ZOODLES & MEATBALLS

MAKES 1 SERVING

691 calories | 54g fat | 8g carbs | 32g protein

3 ounces ground beef chuck

3 ounces ground pork

Sea salt and pepper, to taste

Dried parsley, to taste

Onion powder, to taste

1 ounce pork rinds, crushed

1 large egg, beaten

1 tablespoon olive oil

5 ounces zucchini, spiralized

¼ teaspoon minced garlic

⅓ cup low-carb marinara sauce

Preheat the oven to 400 degrees Fahrenheit, and line a baking sheet with foil or parchment paper; then set it aside.

Combine the beef and pork in a medium bowl, break them up into smaller chunks, add seasonings, and continue to combine.

Add the crushed pork rinds and the egg. Mix with your hands until everything is combined very well.

Roll meat into 6 meatballs.

Place the meatballs on the prepared baking sheet. Bake the meatballs for 15 to 20 minutes.

Meanwhile, drizzle the olive oil in a small skillet over medium heat, add the zucchini and garlic, and season to taste with salt and pepper. Sauté until the zucchini is bright green and just soft, about 5 minutes.

While the zucchini is cooking, heat up the low-carb marinara.

Place the meatballs on top of the zucchini, top with the marinara, and enjoy.

KETO

VEGAN/
VEGETARIAN
RECIPES

BERRY BREAKFAST BOWL

MAKES 1 SERVING

622 calories | 50g fat | 28g carbs | 24g protein (14g net carbs)

½ cup coconut milk, from a can

3 tablespoons hemp hearts

¼ teaspoon vanilla extract

1 tablespoon chia seeds

2 tablespoons flaxseed meal

Stevia, to taste

¼ cup walnuts

¼ cup raspberries

¼ cup blueberries

Combine the coconut milk, hemp hearts, vanilla extract, chia seeds, flaxseed, and stevia in a mason jar, and put it in the refrigerator overnight. This will make it thicken.

The next morning, when you're ready to consume it, spoon the mixture into a bowl and top with the walnuts and berries. Mix and enjoy!

BERRY PROTEIN SHAKE

MAKES 1 SERVING

750 calories | 59g fat | 28g carbs | 28g protein (18g net carbs)

1 cup coconut milk, from a can

1½ scoops vegan vanilla protein powder

1 scoop Complete Wellness Vanilla C8 MCT oil powder

½ medium avocado

¼ cup blueberries

¼ cup raspberries

¼ cup strawberries

Stevia, to taste

Ice, as desired

Place all the ingredients in a blender, and blend until smooth. Pour into a glass and enjoy!

BROCCOLI SLAW SALAD

MAKES 1 SERVING

723 calories | 62g fat | 30g carbs | 21g protein (15g net carbs)

2 cups broccoli slaw

3 tablespoons hemp hearts

½ medium avocado, diced

10 kalamata olives

FOR THE DRESSING:

2 tablespoons tahini

1 teaspoon minced garlic

1 tablespoon extra-virgin olive oil

1 teaspoon lemon juice

Sea salt and pepper, to taste

Combine all the ingredients for the dressing in a small bowl and set it aside.

Layer the broccoli slaw, hemp hearts, avocado, and olives in a large bowl. Drizzle with the salad dressing, and toss until well coated. Enjoy!

BROCCOLI STIR-FRY

MAKES 1 SERVING

635 calories | 47g fat | 22g carbs | 28g protein (11g net carbs)

1½ cups chopped broccoli

¼ medium red pepper, chopped

1 tablespoon avocado oil

4 ounces tofu

3 tablespoons natural peanut butter

¼ teaspoon sesame oil

¼ teaspoon coconut aminos

½ teaspoon chili paste

1 teaspoon apple cider vinegar

½ tablespoon sesame seeds

Cut the broccoli and pepper into small pieces, and set aside.

Put the avocado oil and tofu in a large wok. Fry until lightly browned.

Add the peanut butter, sesame oil, coconut aminos, chili paste, and vinegar to the wok with the tofu and sauté.

Remove half the sauce into a small dish and set aside.

Then add the broccoli and peppers to the tofu mixture, sautéing for 2 to 3 minutes or until the broccoli is bright green.

Remove the stir-fry from the pan and plate. Top with the remaining sauce and with the sesame seeds.

CHOCOLATE PEANUT BUTTER SHAKE

MAKES 1 SERVING

572 calories | 43g fat | 25g carbs | 34g protein (11g net carbs)

12 ounces unsweetened almond milk

1½ scoops vegan chocolate protein powder

1 tablespoon coconut oil

1 cup fresh spinach

2 tablespoons natural peanut butter

1 tablespoon unsweetened cacao powder

Stevia, to taste

Ice, as desired

Place all the ingredients in a blender, and blend until smooth. Enjoy!

VEGETARIANS:
Reduce protein powder to 1 scoop, blend all ingredients, and enjoy with 2 hard-boiled eggs on the side.

CHOCOLATE STRAWBERRY PROTEIN SMOOTHIE

MAKES 1 SERVING

676 calories | 55g fat | 16g carbs | 29g protein (9g net carbs)

1 cup coconut milk, from a can

¼ cup frozen strawberries

3 tablespoons hemp hearts

1 tablespoon unsweetened cacao powder

1 scoop vanilla or chocolate vegan protein powder

Stevia, to taste

Ice, as desired

Put the ingredients in a blender, and blend until smooth. Enjoy!

CREAMY BROCCOLI SOUP

MAKES 1 SERVING

651 calories | 48g fat | 31g carbs | 25g protein (16g net carbs)

1 cup vegetable stock

½ teaspoon minced garlic

3 tablespoons minced onion

½ tablespoon coconut oil

10½ ounces broccoli, cut into florets

¼ cup coconut milk, from a can

Sea salt and pepper, to taste

1 tablespoon coconut cream

½ teaspoon extra-virgin olive oil

3 tablespoons hemp hearts

2 tablespoons sunflower seeds

3 tablespoons unsweetened toasted coconut flakes

Simmer the vegetable stock in a large pot over low to medium heat until it's reduced by at least half.

Meanwhile, sauté the garlic and onions in a skillet in ¼ tablespoon of coconut oil.

When the stock is reduced, remove from the heat and add the broccoli. Cover and allow it to sit for 10 to 12 minutes.

Place the pot back on the heat and add coconut milk, sautéed onion and garlic mix, salt, and pepper, and cook for 2 minutes or until heated.

Transfer the soup to a blender or food processor, and blend until smooth. Add the coconut cream and remaining ¼ tablespoon coconut oil.

Place the soup in a bowl and top with olive oil, hemp hearts, sunflower seeds, and coconut flakes. Enjoy!

GREEK SALAD

678 calories | 57g fat | 18g carbs | 21g protein (12g net carbs)

3 ounces tofu, cubed

½ tablespoon olive oil

Sea salt and pepper, to taste

Italian seasoning, to taste

2 cups romaine salad mix

6 grape tomatoes

½ cup chopped cucumber

1 tablespoon chopped red onion

6 kalamata olives

3 tablespoons hemp hearts

FOR THE DRESSING:

2 tablespoons extra-virgin olive oil

1 teaspoon lemon juice

1 teaspoon red wine vinegar

¼ teaspoon minced garlic

¼ teaspoon oregano

Sea salt and pepper, to taste

Fry the tofu in olive oil in a skillet, and then season with sea salt, pepper, and Italian seasoning to taste. Fry for 6 to 8 minutes or until the tofu is browned around the edges.

Combine the ingredients for the dressing in a small bowl and set it aside.

Layer the salad mix, tomatoes, cucumber, onion, and olives in a large bowl. Top with tofu, sprinkle with hemp hearts, and drizzle with dressing. Toss to combine well and enjoy!

PAD THAI

MAKES 1 SERVING

470 calories | 33g fat | 30g carbs | 19g protein (19g net carbs)

1 cup shirataki noodles

1 tablespoon coconut oil

1 teaspoon minced garlic

4 ounces tofu

½ cup chopped broccoli

½ cup sliced mushrooms

¼ cup thinly sliced red bell pepper

½ teaspoon crushed red pepper flakes

Sea salt and pepper, to taste

1 green onion, sliced

FOR THE SAUCE:

3 tablespoons coconut aminos

1 tablespoon tahini

1 teaspoon sesame seed oil

Prepare the noodles by draining and rinsing them very well.

Combine the sauce ingredients in a small dish until mixed well.

Place the coconut oil, garlic, tofu, broccoli, mushrooms, and bell pepper in a wok over medium heat. Season with the red pepper flakes, sea salt, and pepper. Sauté until the broccoli is bright green and the bell pepper is just soft, about 5 to 7 minutes. Remove from wok and set aside.

Add the noodles and sauce to the same wok, and toss until the noodles are well coated. Add the vegetable mixture back in and cook for 1 minute, stirring the whole time.

Remove from heat and plate. Top with sliced green onion and enjoy!

PEANUT BUTTER NO OATS OATMEAL

MAKES 1 SERVING

813 calories | 65g fat | 27g carbs | 35g protein (17g net carbs)

1 tablespoon flaxseeds, crushed

⅓ cup almond meal

3 tablespoons unsweetened shredded coconut

½ scoop vegan vanilla protein powder

2 tablespoons hemp seeds

1 scoop Complete Wellness Vanilla C8 MCT Oil Powder

Stevia, to taste

¼ teaspoon vanilla extract

½ cup unsweetened almond milk

2 tablespoons natural peanut butter, melted

Grind the flaxseeds in a coffee or spice grinder.

Combine the dry ingredients in a saucepan. Add the wet ingredients, except for the peanut butter, and mix well to combine.

Heat over medium heat, stirring continuously for about 5 minutes or until thick.

Place in a bowl and drizzle melted peanut butter on top. Enjoy!

PORTOBELLO MUSHROOM SALAD
WITH LEMON POPPY SEED DRESSING

MAKES 1 SERVING

754 calories | 67g fat | 20g carbs | 20g protein (11g net carbs)

½ tablespoon avocado oil

½ cup chopped portobello mushrooms

Sea salt and pepper, to taste

½ cup shredded cabbage

4 cups power greens salad mix

3 tablespoons hemp hearts

1 tablespoon chopped walnuts

FOR THE DRESSING:

2½ tablespoons avocado oil

⅛ cup lemon juice

½ teaspoon ground ginger

Sea salt and pepper, to taste

1½ tablespoons poppy seeds

For the dressing, place all the ingredients in a mason jar or a container with a lid and shake well to combine.

Put ½ tablespoon of avocado oil and mushrooms in a small skillet and season with sea salt and pepper. Sauté until the mushrooms are just soft, about 5 minutes.

In a large bowl, layer the cabbage, salad mix, mushrooms, hemp hearts, and walnuts. Drizzle with the dressing, and toss until evenly coated. Enjoy!

SPRING ROLL BOWL

MAKES 1 SERVING

641 calories | 48g fat | 28g carbs | 21g protein (24g net carbs)

3 ounces tofu, cubed

2 cups shredded cabbage

½ cup sliced zucchini

½ cup sliced red pepper

1 green onion, chopped

FOR THE DRESSING:

1 tablespoon stevia

2 tablespoons avocado oil

1½ tablespoons coconut aminos

2½ tablespoons apple cider vinegar

1 clove garlic

2 tablespoons natural peanut butter

Combine all the ingredients for the dressing in a small bowl, and set it aside.

Put tofu and half the dressing in a skillet over medium heat. Fry until the tofu is lightly browned and warmed through, about 5 to 8 minutes.

Add the remaining ingredients, except for the green onion, and the remainder of the dressing to the same skillet. Sauté until the cabbage is wilted and the vegetables are just soft. Allow to cool a few minutes, sprinkle with green onion, and enjoy.

ZUCCHINI PESTO

MAKES 1 SERVING

644 calories | 55g fat | 17g carbs | 27g protein (8g net carbs)

2 tablespoons extra-virgin olive oil

1 clove garlic

2 cups fresh basil

6 tablespoons hemp hearts, divided

2 cups zoodles (zucchini, spiralized)

For the pesto, place the olive oil, garlic, basil, and 4 tablespoons hemp hearts in a blender or food processor, and blend until smooth. Set aside.

Put zoodles and pesto in a skillet over medium heat. Sauté for 1 to 2 minutes and top with remaining hemp hearts. Enjoy!

ZUCCHINI SAGE PASTA

MAKES 1 SERVING

713 calories | 62g fat | 16g carbs | 28g protein (9g net carbs)

1 tablespoon coconut oil

5 ounces tofu, cubed

¼ teaspoon nutmeg

1 tablespoon sage

Sea salt and pepper, to taste

2 tablespoons avocado oil

½ cup chopped broccoli

1 cup spinach

2 cups zoodles

3 tablespoons hemp hearts

Place the coconut oil, tofu, nutmeg, ½ tablespoon sage, sea salt, and pepper in a wok over medium heat. Fry the tofu until its edges just begin to brown, and then set it aside.

Add the avocado oil, the remaining ½ tablespoon sage, and the other remaining ingredients, except for the hemp hearts, to the same wok, and toss until well combined. Sauté until the broccoli is just soft and bright green.

Place zoodles and veggies in a bowl, top with tofu, and sprinkle with the hemp hearts. Enjoy!

KETO

HIGH-CARB RECIPES FOR CYCLICAL KETO DIET

*Note that these are not keto recipes—they are high-carb recipe suggestions for rotating in on the Cyclical Keto Diet discussed in Part 4.

CHICKEN & RICE

MAKES 1 SERVING

569 calories | 20g fat | 57g carbs | 38g protein

1 tablespoon avocado oil

3½-ounce chicken breast, diced

Garlic and herb seasoning, to taste

Sea salt and pepper, to taste

¼ cup chicken gravy

1 cup white rice, cooked

1½ cups broccoli, steamed

Put the avocado oil, chicken breast, and seasonings in a wok over medium heat. Toss the chicken until well coated, and then sauté until the chicken is white and cooked through, about 6 to 8 minutes. Set it aside.

Prepare the chicken gravy according to package instructions.

Layer the rice and gravy on a plate, and top it with the chicken. Enjoy it with steamed broccoli on the side, seasoned with sea salt and pepper.

PEANUT BUTTER PROTEIN WAFFLES

WAFFLE RECIPE MAKES 5 WAFFLES, 1 WAFFLE PER SERVING

Nutrition information with sides: 481 calories | 21g fat | 41g carbs | 37g protein

Nutrition information for 1 waffle: 205 calories | 5g fat | 26g carbs | 18g protein

1 cup whole wheat pastry flour

2 scoops (½ cup) vanilla protein powder

½ cup powdered peanut butter

4 teaspoons baking powder

2 eggs

1 teaspoon vanilla extract

½ cup unsweetened applesauce

1¾ cups unsweetened almond milk

FOR SIDES:

2 eggs

Sea salt and pepper, to taste

½ banana, sliced

¼ cup sugar-free maple syrup

2 slices bacon, cooked

Preheat a Belgian waffle iron.

Mix all the dry ingredients in a large bowl until well combined, and set aside.

Beat together the eggs and vanilla in a small bowl until fluffy.

Mix the egg and vanilla mixture into the dry ingredients. Add the applesauce and milk and mix until well blended and a batter forms. Allow batter to rest for 5 minutes.

Spray the waffle iron with nonstick cooking spray, and pour about ½ cup batter into the waffle iron. Cook according to the manufacturer's instructions.

Meanwhile, spray a skillet with nonstick cooking spray, and fry the eggs to desired doneness. Season with sea salt and pepper.

Top 1 waffle with the sliced banana and sugar-free syrup, and enjoy with the eggs and bacon on the side!

PINEAPPLE SHRIMP MEXI-SALAD

MAKES 1 SERVING

525 calories | 11g fat | 60g carbs | 40g protein

4 ounces shrimp (tails and veins removed)

½ cup pineapple chunks

1 tablespoon lime juice

½ tablespoon honey

¼ teaspoon garlic powder

Pinch of onion powder

¼ teaspoon chili powder

Pinch of red pepper flakes (optional)

½ cup low-sodium black beans, rinsed and drained

3 cups romaine salad mix

¼ cup pico de gallo

⅓ medium avocado, chopped

1 tablespoon sour cream

2 tablespoons salsa

Place the shrimp, pineapple, lime juice, honey, and seasonings in a large frying pan or wok over medium heat. Stir until the shrimp is evenly coated, and then add black beans.

Sauté until the shrimp is pink and curling in, about 8 minutes. Remove from the heat and allow to cool.

Meanwhile, layer the salad mix, pico de gallo, and avocado in a large bowl. Add the shrimp mixture and sour cream, and drizzle with salsa. Enjoy immediately.

RESOURCES

Drew's Social Media

Instagram: Fit2Fat2Fit

Facebook: Fit2Fat2Fit

Twitter: Fit2Fat2Fit

YouTube: Fit2Fat2Fit

Website

Fit2fat2fit.com

Facebook Support Group

Keeping it Keto

https://www.facebook.com
/groups/1414503145234610

Keto-Friendly Products

Complete Wellness Supplements:
shop.completewellness.com

Nui cookies - eatnui.com

Drop an F Bomb - dropanfbomb.com

Phat Fudge - phatfudge.com

Top 10 Keto Podcasts

The Livin' La Vida Low-Carb Show with Jimmy Moore

The Model Health Show with Shawn Stevenson

The Fat Burning Man Show with Abel James

The Keto Diet Podcast with Leanne Vogel

The Keto Answers Podcast with Dr. Anthony Gustin

Aubrey Marcus Podcast

Dr. Berg's Healthy Keto and Intermittent Fast Podcast

Keto Talk with Jimmy Moore & Dr. Will Cole

Primal Blueprint Podcast with Mark Sisson

Bulletproof Radio with Dave Asprey

And check out my podcast, The Fit2Fat2Fit Experience, on ITunes, Stitcher, Spotify, TuneIn, and iHeart Radio: http://www.fit2fat2fit.com/podcast/

Keto-Centered Fit2Fat2Fit Podcast Episodes

Episode 019: Jimmy Moore and Drew Talk about Ketosis and the Fit2Fat2Fit Docu-Series

Episode 031: Will Adapting to a Ketogenic Diet Help Athletes Work Out More Efficiently? with Dr. Dom D'Agostino

Episode 039: Brain-Focused Smart Drugs, Ketosis, and Old School Style Bodybuilding

Episode 063: You Are What You Eat; So Eat Lard!

Episode 066: The Common Myths and Real Benefits of Fasting

Episode 070: You Don't Have to Suffer through Sobriety

Episode 086: Embrace the Fat!

Episode 090: Nutritional Ketogenics 101

Episode 092: Salt: The Controversial Nutrient

Episode 094: The Real Science Behind a Ketogenic Diet and Lifestyle

Episode 102: Keto Science

Episode 103: How Keto Can Take Your Body to a Whole New Level of Fitness

Episode 104: How Do You Measure for Ketosis?

Episode 105: Intermittent Fasting: Understanding the Protocols and Debunking the Myths

Episode 113: Can a Ketogenic Diet Help Kill Cancer Cells? with Dr. Adrienne Scheck

Episode 115: Everything You Ever Wanted to Know about Fasting

Favorite Apps

For tracking macros: MyFitnessPal

For meditation: Headspace, Calm, Brain.fm, Insight Timer

Gratitude journal: 5 Minute Journal, Uplifter

Favorite Books

Daring Greatly by Brené Brown

Rising Strong by Brené Brown

Braving the Wilderness by Brené Brown

Loving What Is by Byron Katie

The Art of Living by Bob Proctor

You Are a Badass by Jen Sincero

Ego Is the Enemy by Ryan Holiday

The Obstacle Is the Way by Ryan Holiday

The Four Agreements by Don Miguel Ruiz

The Fifth Agreement by Don Miguel Ruiz

Talking to Your Doctor or Other Care Provider about Keto

It's always a good idea to talk to your doctor about any changes to your diet and lifestyle, so I recommend you do so when starting keto. But what if your doctor is resistant to the keto diet?

First, keep in mind that your relationship with your doctor should be one of mutual respect. Too often we feel they're the experts and they have the final say. They don't get to control you, but at the same time you don't always want to be fighting with everything they recommend or prescribe—it should be a give-and-take between you, as an expert on yourself, and your care provider, as an experienced, hopefully well-read medical professional. Sometimes what you need is to see a different doctor, someone who listens to you! But sometimes what you need is to have a good in-depth conversation.

So if you're having trouble talking keto with your doctor, go in to your next appointment with this book and some of the many published pieces on the ketogenic diet—studies on keto span almost 20 years and feature peer-reviewed (the gold standard in academic and scientific publications) reports on keto showing improvements in cognitive function and mental clarity and reductions in complications resulting from high cholesterol, diabetes, epilepsy, Parkinson's, Alzheimer's, and even cancer. Point to evidence and show that you're doing your homework. Let them know that this isn't a fad diet; it's been around for a while, it's been well studied, and it's been used for therapeutic purposes by the medical community for a long time. Even ask if your doctor would be willing to do some reading about keto.

Ask for specifics if your doctor has concerns: what are they concerned about? That way, you can do your own research and see if there's an answer to their questions, which you can discuss together. Ask about supplements and interactions with any of your medications as well.

The bottom line: do your research and ask questions. It's your health, and when you take the initiative to partner with your doctor, you'll avoid the negative effects of being passive with your new fitness-oriented lifestyle. You deserve a care provider who is willing to listen to you.

Being skeptical about keto is okay, whether the skeptic is you or your doctor. Better to ask questions, educate yourself, and have a good conversation with your doctor so that when you begin your keto journey you are embracing a new you with integrity and confidence.

ENDNOTES

Introduction

1. Brené Brown, "Own Our History. Change the Story" (blog), June 18, 2015, https://brenebrown.com/blog/2015/06/18/own-our-history-change-the-story/.

Part 1

1. Mahshid Dehghan, Andrew Mente, Xiaohe Zhang, et al., "Associations of Fats and Carbohydrate Intake with Cardiovascular Disease and Mortality in 18 Countries from Five Continents (PURE): A Prospective Cohort Study," *The Lancet* 309, no. 10107 (November 2017): 2050–2062.

2. Leading M.D. and researcher Eric Westman finds that "eating a ketogenic diet lowers inflammation naturally, without the use of prescription medications such as statins. It's this inflammation that is the true culprit in heart disease, and the fact that ketosis reduces systemic inflammation is further evidence supporting the use of a low-carb, high-fat diet for improving heart health." Jimmy Moore with Eric C. Westman, M.D., *Keto Clarity: Your Definitive Guide to the Benefits of a Low-Carb, High-Fat Diet* (Las Vegas, NV: Victory Belt Publishing, 2014). See also H. M. Dashti, T. C. Mathew, T. Hussein, et al., "Long-Term Effects of a Ketogenic Diet in Obese Patients," *Experimental & Clinical Cardiology* 9, no. 3 (2004): 200–205. This study of the long-term effects of the ketogenic diet found that "a high fat diet rich in polyunsaturated fatty acids (ketogenic diet) is quite effective in reducing body weight and the risk factors for various chronic diseases."

3. Allison Aubrey, "What the Industry Knew about Sugar's Health Effects, But Didn't Tell Us," NPR, November 21, 2017, https://www.npr.org/sections/thesalt/2017/11/21/565766988/what-the-industry-knew-about-sugars-health-effects-but-didnt-tell-us.

4. The Organisation for Economic Co-operation and Development (OECD), Obesity Update 2017, http://www.oecd.org/health/obesity-update.htm, accessed February 21, 2018.

5. Moore and Westman, *Keto Clarity*.

6. M. Guzmán and C. Blázquez, "Ketone Body Synthesis in the Brain: Possible Neuroprotective Effects," *Prostaglandins, Leukotrienes, and Essential Fatty Acids* 70, no. 3 (March 2004): 287–292. See also Mark Sission, "How Much Glucose Does Your Brain Really Need?" *Mark's Daily Apple* (blog), July 2, 2012, https://www.marksdailyapple.com/how-much-glucose-does-your-brain-really-need/.

7. Hussein M. Dasht, Thazhumpal C. Mathew, Talib Hussein, et al., "Long-Term Effects of a Ketogenic Diet in Obese Patients," *Experimental and Clinical Cardiology* 9, no. 3 (Fall 2004): 200–205.

8. P. Barbanti, L. Fofi, et al., "Ketogenic Diet in Migraine: Rationale, Findings and Perspectives," *Neurological Sciences* 38, suppl 1 (May 2017): 111–115.

9. M. M. Villaluz, L. B. Lomax, et al., "The Ketogenic Diet Is Effective for Refractory Epilepsy Associated with Acquired Structural Epileptic Encephalopathy," *Developmental Medicine and Child Neurology* 60, no. 7 (July 2018): 718–723; Emmanuelle C. S. Bostock, Kenneth C. Kirkby, et al., "The Current Status of the Ketogenic Diet in Psychiatry," *Frontiers in Psychiatry* 8, no. 43 (2017), http://doi.org/10.3389/fpsyt.2017.00043; B. C. Perng, M. Chen, et al., "A Keto-Mediet Approach with Coconut Substitution and Exercise May Delay the Onset of Alzheimer's Disease among Middle-Aged," *The Journal of Prevention of Alzheimer's Disease* 4, no. 1 (2017): 51–57; and C. Veyrat-Durebex, P. Reynier, et al., "How Can a Ketogenic Diet Improve Motor Function?" *Frontiers in Molecular Neuroscience* 11, no. 15 (January 2018).

10. T. Walczyk and J. Y. Wick, "The Ketogenic Diet: Making a Comeback," *The Consultant Pharmacist* 32, no. 7 (July 2017): 388–396; and Mithu Storoni and Gordon T. Plant, "The Therapeutic Potential of the Ketogenic Diet in Treating Progressive Multiple Sclerosis," *Multiple Sclerosis International*, published online December 29, 2015.

11. R. S. El-Mallakh and M. E. Paskitti, "The Ketogenic Miet May Have Mood-Stabilizing Properties," *Medical Hypotheses* 57, no. 6 (December 2001): 724–726.

12. E. C. Westman, W. S. Yancy, Jr., M. K. Olsen, et al., "Effect of a Low-Carbohydrate, Ketogenic Diet Program Compared to a Low-Fat Diet on Fasting Lipoprotein Subclasses," *International Journal of Cardiology* 110, no. 2 (June 16, 2006): 212–216.

13. Joseph Mercola, "The Cholesterol Myth That Is Harming Your Health," Mercola.com, August 10, 2010, https://articles.mercola.com/sites/articles/archive/2010/08/10/making-sense-of-your-cholesterol-numbers.aspx.

14. D. A. Fomin, B. McDaniel, et al., "The Promising Potential Role of Ketones in Inflammatory Dermatologic Disease: A New Frontier in Treatment Research," *The Journal of Dermatological Treatment* 28, no. 6 (September 2017): 484–487.

15. Hormones that affect weight loss: insulin, GLP-1, OXM, Apo-AIV, glucagon, ghrelin,

leptin, PP, adiponectin, enterostatin, amylin, somatostatin, neurotensin, neurotrophic factor, CRH, TRH, alpha-MSH, MCH, NPY, AgRP, GABA, TSH, T3, T4, peptid YY, cholecystikinin, ghrelin, gastric inhibitory peptide, and pancreatic polypeptide. Estrogen, progesterone, and testosterone are all steroid hormones made from cholesterol. Consumption of healthy saturated fats (coconut oil and fatty meats) helps naturally increase these, whereas unhealthy fats like vegetable oil lower these hormones.

16. C. Wright and N. L. Simone, "Obesity and Tumor Growth: Inflammation, Immunity, and the Role of a Ketogenic Diet," *Current Opinion in Clinical Nutrition and Metabolic Care* 19, no. 4 (July 2016): 294–299.

17. A. Goday, D. Bellido, I. Sajoux, et al., "Short-Term Safety, Tolerability and Efficacy of a Very Low-Calorie-Ketogenic Diet Interventional Weight Loss Program versus Hypocaloric Diet in Patients with Type 2 Diabetes Mellitus," *Nutrition & Diabetes* 6, no. 9 (September 19, 2016).

18. A. Paoli, K. Grimaldi, L. Toniolo, et al., "Nutrition and Acne: Therapeutic Potential of Ketogenic Diets," *Skin Pharmacology and Physiology* 25, no. 3 (2012): 111–117.

19. Westin Childs, "6 Causes of High Testosterone in Women and How to Lower Your Levels" (blog), accessed on August 9, 2018, https://www.restartmed.com /high-testosterone-women/; and G. U. Liepa, A. Sengupta, et al., "Polycystic Ovary Syndrome (PCOS) and Other Androgen Excess-Related Conditions: Can Changes in Dietary Intake Make a Difference?" *Nutrition*
in Clinical Practice* 23, no. 1 (February 2008): 63–71.

20. J. C. Mavropoulos, W. S. Yancy, J. Hepburn, et al., "The Effects of a Low-Carbohydrate, Ketogenic Diet on the Polycystic Ovary Syndrome: a Pilot Study," *Nutrition & Metabolism* 2, no. 35 (December 2005). In this study, two out of five women became pregnant after 24 weeks of living ketogenic and improved hormones.

Part 2

1. A. C. Famurewa, C. A. Ekeleme-Egedigwe, S. C. Nwali, et al., "Dietary Supplementation with Virgin Coconut Oil Improves Lipid Profile and Hepatic Antioxidant Status and Has Potential Benefits on Cardiovascular Risk Indices in Normal Rats," *Journal of Dietary Supplements* 15, no. 3 (May 4, 2018): 330–342; and S. K. Yeap, B. K. Beh, N. M. Ali, et al., "Antistress and Antioxidant Effects of Virgin Coconut Oil *In Vivo*," *Experimental and Therapeutic Medicine* 9, no. 1 (January 2015): 39–42.

2. Dominic D'Agostino, "Ketone Supplements May Help Reduce Anxiety" (blog), March 15, 2017, https://dominicdagostino.wordpress .com/2017/03/15/ketone-supplements-may- help-reduce-anxiety/.

3. M. Goyal, S. Singh, E. M. Sibinga, et al., "Meditation Programs for Psychological Stress and Well-Being: A Systematic Review and Meta-analysis," *JAMA Internal Medicine* 174, no. 3 (March 2014): 357–368. doi: 10.1001/jamainternmed.2013.13018; and Melissa A. Rosenkranz, Richard J. Davidson,

Donal G. MacCoon, et al., "A Comparison of Mindfulness-Based Stress Reduction and an Active Control in Modulation of Neurogenic Inflammation," *Brain, Behavior, and Immunity* 27 (January 2013): 174–184, http://www.sciencedirect.com/science/article/pii/S0889159112004758.

4.   J. Martires and M. Zeidler, "The Value of Mindfulness Meditation in the Treatment of Insomnia," *Current Opinion in Pulmonary Medicine* 21, no. 6 (November 2015): 547–552; T. Gard, B. K. Hölzel, and S. W. Lazar, "The Potential Effects of Meditation on Age-Related Cognitive Decline: A Systematic Review," *Annals of the New York Academy of Science* 1307 (January 2014): 89–103; and A. J. Lang, J. L. Strauss, J. Bomyea, et al., "The Theoretical and Empirical Basis for Meditation as an Intervention for PTSD," *Behavior Modification* 36, no. 6 (November 2012): 759–786.

Part 3

1.   "Lactose Intolerance," Genetics Home Reference, U.S. National Library of Medicine, May 8, 2018, https://ghr.nlm.nih.gov/condition/lactose-intolerance#statistics.

2.   M. P. Mattson and R. Wan, "Beneficial Effects of Intermittent Fasting and Caloric Restriction on the Cardiovascular and Cerebrovascular Systems," *Journal of Nutritional Biochemistry* 16, no. 3 (March 2005): 129–137.

3.   M. Wei et al., "Fasting-Mimicking Diet and Markers/Risk Factors for Aging, Diabetes, Cancer, and Cardiovascular Disease," *Science Translational Medicine* 9, no. 377 (February 2015); and Megumi Hatori et al., "Time-Restricted Feeding without Reducing Caloric Intake Prevents Metabolic Diseases in Mice Fed a High-Fat Diet," *Cell Metabolism* 15, no. 6 (June 6, 2012): 848–860, https://www.cell.com/cell-metabolism/fulltext/S1550-4131(12)00189-1.

4.   Jason Fung, "Fasting and Lipolysis, Part 4," *Intensive Dietary Management*, https://idmprogram.com/fasting-and-lipolysis-part-4/, accessed at on May 9, 2018.

5.   Mattson and Wan, "Beneficial Effects of Intermittent Fasting and Caloric Restriction on the Cardiovascular and Cerebrovascular Systems."

6.   W. K. Stewart and L. Fleming, "Features of a Successful Therapeutic Fast of 382 Days' Duration," *Postgraduate Medical Journal* 49 (March 1973): 203–209.

INDEX

NOTE:

The term *veg*n* stands for "vegan" and "vegetarian."
Page numbers in *italics* indicate recipes.

Greens, powdered, 58

Grilled Chicken Thighs with Sautéed Cauliflower Medley, *281*

Grilled Rib Eye & Asparagus, *282*

Guacamole Burger with Bacon-Wrapped Asparagus Stacks, *285*

H

Heart health and disease, 6–7, 12

Hormones, balancing, 12, 23, 64–65, 82, 83, 150

I

Inflammation
carbohydrates and, 6
dairy quality and, 60–61, 81
disease correlation, xiv, 6, 7, 12
exogenous ketones helping with, 59
ketogenic diet reducing, xiv, xviii, 6, 7, 12
meditation helping, 72
nuts and, 81–82
unhealthy fats causing, 48, 60, 81

Ingredients. *See also specific main ingredients*
Complete Keto must-haves, 90
grocery and pantry lists for Weeks 1 to 4, 91, 100, 108, 117

Intentions/goals, publicly announcing, 25–26

Intermittent Keto Diet, 137–138, 147–148

Intuitive eating, 150

Italian restaurants, keto and eating at, 63

J

Jambalaya, *286*

Jerk Chicken & Veggie Kabobs, *289*

Journal, keeping, 27, 46, 47, 73

Juices, saying no to, 54

Jumping squats, 165

K

Kabobs, chicken and veggie, *289*

Ketoacidosis, 10

Keto-adapted, ketosis vs., 42–43

Keto Chicken Chow Mein, *290*

Keto Cobb Salad, *221*

Keto flu, 60, 65

Keto Flu Killer (Drew's Homemade Electrolyte Drink), *182*

Keto for life, 135–155
about: moving on from CK30, 135–137
benefits and popularity of keto lifestyle, 11–12
choosing between diet approaches, 137–139
Cyclical Keto Diet and, 137–138, 144–147. *See also* Recipes, high-carb for Cyclical Keto Diet
extended fasting and, 141
Intermittent Keto Diet and, 137–138, 147–148
long-term emotional challenge hacks, 149–153
roadmap for success, 153–155
self-sufficiency and, 135–137
staying in keto long-term, 138–139

taking off the training wheels analogy, 135–136
Targeted Keto Diet and, 137–138, 142–144
testing for ketosis long-term, 148–149
troubleshooting guidelines, 140

Ketogenic diet. *See also* Dos and don'ts; Ketosis; Starting diet
alcohol and, 68–69
Atkins diet and, 8–9
benefits of, xiii–xv, 11–12
as body's backup system, 4
consulting doctor before beginning, xviii, 329
defined, 2–5
emotional obstacle to avoid, 35–37
finding your "why" for doing, xix, 24–25
foods to avoid, 19–20
foods to eat, 16–19
ketoacidosis and, 10
for life. *See* Keto for life
myths about. *See* Myths about keto
Paleo diet and, 2–5
protein intake and, 8–9
purpose of, 2
safety of, 9–10
side effects, 60–61
testimonials. *See* Testimonials and "before" and "after" photos
time for body to adjust to, 4–5
tips and tricks. *See* Dos and don'ts

Keto Hot Chocolate, *183*

Keto lifestyle. *See* Keto for life

Ketones. *See also* Ketosis

fat intake clogs arteries, increases heart disease, 6–7

gallbladder is required for keto, 10

ketoacidosis is linked to keto diet, 10

keto causes muscle loss, 9

keto is just Atkins repackaged, 8–9

long-term keto is not safe, 9–10

N

Nutrition labels, reading, 47

Nuts
about: almond butter for diet, 21; approved foods list, 127; CK30 plan and, 19; inflammation from, 81; for keto diet, 19; keto diet and, 22, 81; reintroducing after CK30, 19, 142; veg*n diet and, 22

Berry Breakfast Bowl, *308*

Chocolate Peanut Butter Shake, *312*

Peanut Butter No Oats Oatmeal, *317*

Peanut Butter Protein Waffles, *325*

O

Oats, lack of nutrients in, 53. *See also* Peanut Butter No Oats Oatmeal

Obesity, fat intake and, 6–7

Oils, best sources of, 17, 21

Onions, caramelizing precaution, 48

P

Pad Thai, *316*

Paleo Mayo, *184*

Paleo Ranch Dressing, *185*

Pancakes, *210, 225*

Parkinson's disease, keto and, 11, 329

Parties, keto and, 62

Pasta and zoodles
about: lack of nutrients in pasta, 54

Chicken Artichoke Zoodle Pan, *265*

Pad Thai, *316*

Zoodles & Meatballs, *305*

Zucchini Sage Pasta, *321*

Pastas, avoiding, 50

PCOS (Polycystic Ovarian Syndrome), 12, 23, 157

Peanut Butter No Oats Oatmeal, *317*

Peanut Butter Protein Waffles, *325*

Peppers, unstuffed, *302*

Perfection
Amy's story, 35–37

antidote for striving for, 37–39

dining out, travel and, 64

Lauren's story, 79–80

pressuring yourself with, 35–37, 79–80

self-experimentation instead of, 80

self-forgiveness and, 37, 80, 81

Pesto, zucchini, *320*

Phase one. *See* CK30 (Complete Keto 30); CK30 day-by-day "to dos"

Phase two. *See* Keto for life

Pineapple Shrimp Mexi-Salad, *326*

Plank and side plank, 170–171

Plateaus, handling, 116

Polish Sausage with Fried Cabbage & Collard Greens, *294*

Pork. *See also* Sausage
about: best sources of, 17; grocery lists for Weeks 1 to 4, 91, 100, 108, 117

Baked Ranch Pork Chops with Bacon Broccoli, *257*

Dry Rub Ribs & Lemon Garlic Roasted Vegetables, *273*

Meat Lovers' Scramble, *227*

Shredded Pork Salad, *236*

Smoked Chili Pork Chop with Green Beans, *298*

Unstuffed Peppers, *302*

Zoodles & Meatballs, *305*

Portobello Mushroom Salad with Lemon Poppy Seed Dressing, *318*

Positive affirmations, 74–75, 86, 89, 92, 95, 125. *See also* CK30 day-by-day "to dos"

Potassium
levels in foods, 51–53

supplements, 45–46, 57, 59, 60, 88

Poultry. *See* Chicken

Powdered greens, 58

Probiotics and fermented foods, 58

Protein
to eat on keto diet, 17

ACKNOWLEDGMENTS

First and foremost I'd like to thank my two daughters, Kale'a and Kiana, for loving me unconditionally as their dad and for giving me purpose in life. They are my why. Thank you to my ex-wife, Lynn, for being an awesome mom to our daughters and bringing them into this world. I'm so grateful that we've both been able to swallow our pride and maintain a good relationship to give our daughters the best life we can.

Thank you to my 'Ohana, Mom, Dad, and all 10 of my brothers and sisters. All the amazing experiences we've all had together so far in this life have helped shape me into who I am today.

A team of awesome women helped me put this book together: Colleen Martell, my fierce and fearless co-writer, is wicked talented at making my ideas, my voice, and my passion for helping people flow on the page. My agent, Stephanie Tade, is a problem-solving machine and her expertise and

insight improved this book every step of the way. And last but not least, my assistant, Ashtyn Blanchard, worked tirelessly behind the scenes with everything from photography to recipe development. These three are why the book turned out so well.

The entire Hay House team, and in particular my editor Anne Barthel, was so great to work with. Thank you for letting me be me in this book and for your unwavering enthusiasm in delivering my message. This experience has changed my life and your support through this whole process means the world to me.

I'd also like to thank my business partner and good friend, Los Silva, and the entire marketing team in Florida for helping me take my message and content and touch so many more people's lives than I could've ever accomplished by myself. I'm so appreciative of all the hard work that they do behind the scenes.

So many mentors and life coaches have helped me navigate the hard times of my life and I owe a deep debt of gratitude to them. Those hard times have taught me so much and because of the wisdom and authenticity shared by mentors and coaches I've been able to grow the most when times got tough. So in a way, I'm grateful for all the mistakes I've made, because learning from them and growing from them have helped me discover a better version of myself. Life happens for me and not to me.

Thank you to authors Brené Brown, Don Miguel Ruiz, and others whose profound teachings have changed my life in so many ways—I'm grateful that *Daring Greatly, Rising Strong, Braving the Wilderness, The Four Agreements, You Are a Badass, The Art of Living, Ego Is the Enemy, Loving What Is,* and books like these are out there for us to learn from. I've learned so much about guilt, shame, empathy, courage, integrity, and many other lessons from these authors. They've helped me embrace my vulnerability as a strength, own my story, let go of ego, and not take things personally. They've taught me that I'm in charge of my own happiness. Change my perception, change my story, change my life.

Thank you to everyone who has supported and followed me from the early Fit2Fat2Fit years until now. I'm still in awe that this journey has become what it is today, and I couldn't have done it without all the amazing fans who could see my true message in doing this crazy experiment. So thank you for believing in me, trusting me, and allowing me to gain a better understanding in my journey to try to help people.

Keep moving forward: *Imua!*

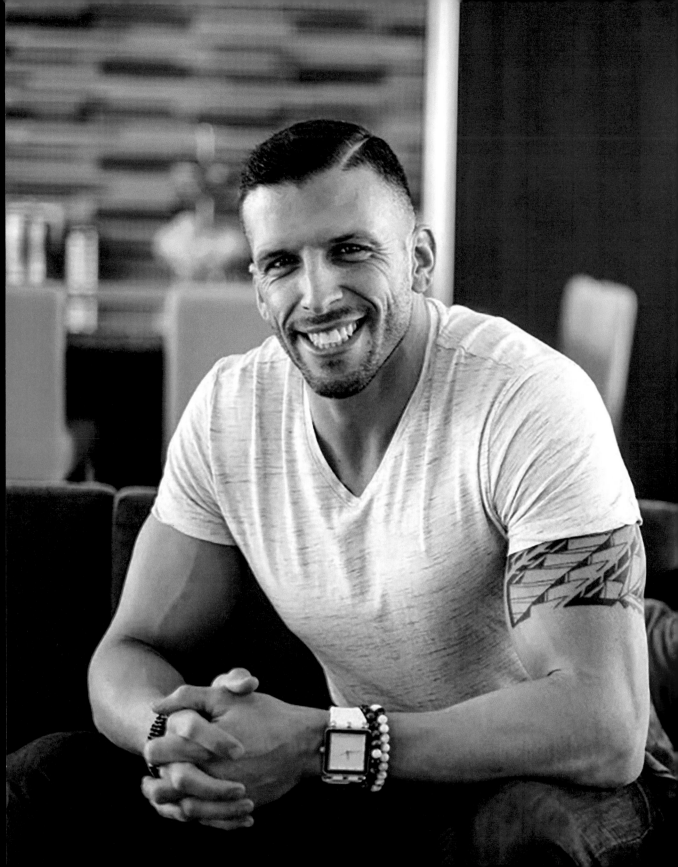

ABOUT THE AUTHOR

Health and fitness expert Drew Manning is the *New York Times* best-selling author of *Fit2Fat2Fit: The Unexpected Lessons from Gaining and Losing 75 lbs on Purpose*, and has for years been a leading voice in the burgeoning keto diet movement. Drew is also the creator of the A&E Show *Fit to Fat to Fit* and the host of *The Fit2Fat2Fit Experience* podcast. With close to a million social media followers, Drew continues to transform people's lives all around the world.

Known for his straightforward and empathetic fitness and health coaching, Drew has been featured on *The Dr. Oz Show*, CNN, *Good Morning America*, *The Tonight Show with Jay Leno*, *The View*, MSNBC, and *Yahoo!*, among other media outlets. Drew's message is that it's not just about weight loss and looking great; it's about living an optimal life. Refusing to take the health and fitness industry as is, Drew is one of the leaders of a movement to change the industry from one that sells an external ideal of perfection to consumers who feel anxious about their weight and their health to one that empowers individuals to find their own best version of themselves.

Through the powerfully transformative keto diet and his own honest and candid personal testimonial, Drew is able to lead people to living optimally and feeling amazing, and through major spiritual, mental, and emotional transformations. His goal is to help people find not just physical success, but internal fulfillment. His message, which resonates with millions of people, is that it's not about the results—it's about finding love and happiness in the process.

Drew lives in Salt Lake City, Utah, with his daughters, who remind him every day not to take things too seriously.

HAY HOUSE TITLES OF RELATED INTEREST

YOU CAN HEAL YOUR LIFE, the movie,
starring Louise Hay & Friends

(available as a 1-DVD program, an expanded 2-DVD set, and an online streaming video)
Learn more at www.hayhouse.com/louise-movie

THE SHIFT, the movie,
starring Dr. Wayne W. Dyer

(available as a 1-DVD program, an expanded 2-DVD set, and an online streaming video)
Learn more at www.hayhouse.com/the-shift-movie

THE ALLERGY SOLUTION:
Unlock the Surprising, Hidden Truth about
Why You Are Sick and How to Get Well,
by Leo Galland, M.D., and Jonathan Galland, J.D.

THE DENTAL DIET:
The Surprising Link between Your Teeth, Real Food,
and Life-Changing Natural Health,
by Dr. Steven Lin

FAT FOR FUEL:
A Revolutionary Diet to Combat Cancer,
Boost Brain Power, and Increase Your Energy,
by Dr. Joseph Mercola

FAT FOR FUEL KETOGENIC COOKBOOK:
Recipes and Ketogenic Keys to Health from a World-Class Doctor
and an Internationally Renowned Chef, by Dr. Joseph Mercola and Pete Evans

All of the above are available at your local bookstore,
or may be ordered by contacting Hay House (see next page).

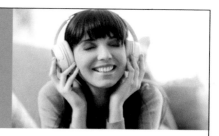

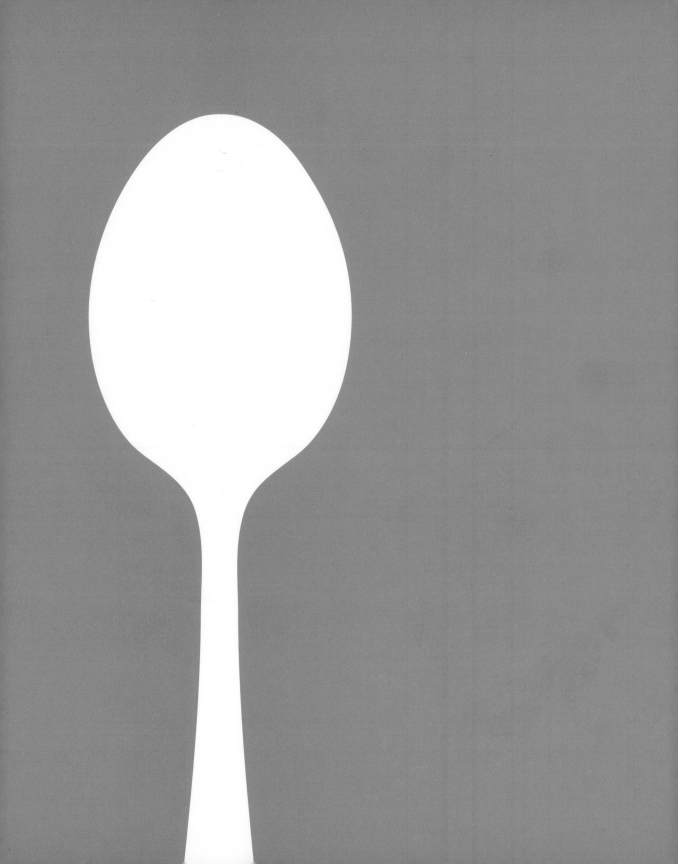